We Can Do Better

Urgent Innovations

to Improve Mental Health

Access and Care

David Goldbloom, M.D.

Published by Simon & Schuster

New York   London   Toronto   Sydney   New Delhi

Simon & Schuster Canada
A Division of Simon & Schuster, Inc.
166 King Street East, Suite 300
Toronto, Ontario M5A 1J3

This Simon & Schuster Canada edition May 2021

SIMON & SCHUSTER CANADA and colophon are
trademarks of Simon & Schuster, Inc.

For information about special discounts for bulk purchases,
please contact Simon & Schuster Special Sales at
1-800-268-3216 or CustomerService@simonandschuster.ca.

Manufactured in the United States of America

1   3   5   7   9   10   8   6   4   2

Library and Archives Canada Cataloguing in Publication
Title: We can do better: urgent innovations to improve mental
health access and care / David Goldbloom.
Names: Goldbloom, David S., author.
Description: Simon & Schuster Canada edition.
Identifiers: Canadiana (print) 20200337378 | Canadiana (ebook) 20200337696
| ISBN 9781501184864 (hardcover) | ISBN 9781501184888 (ebook)
Subjects: LCSH: Mental health services. | LCSH: Mental
health services—Technological innovations.
Classification: LCC RA790.5 .G65 2021 | DDC 362.2—dc23

ISBN 978-1-5011-8486-4
ISBN 978-1-5011-8488-8 (ebook)

To my dedicated colleagues and future generations of them—
all of whom want to do better for people with
mental illnesses and their families

Contents

◇◇◇◇

Contents

WE CAN DO BETTER

Foreword

◇◇◇◇

This foreword began with a curious bargain. David Goldbloom contacted me to ask if I would write something for his latest book. I was about to accept with alacrity. I had fond memories of reading David's previous book, *How Can I Help?: A Week in My Life as a Psychiatrist*. It was inspirational and a guiding beacon for my wife, Sharon, during her seven years at Rideau Hall, where her major public priority was to illuminate mental health awareness and care across the land. But then came the sober second thought. I recalled, with a chuckle, that I have never had a conversation with David without some laughter and usually a joke.

So I reminded David that while he was board chair of the Stratford Festival I had gladly accepted his invitation to join the board. Word has it that the minutes of my first board meeting duly recorded with pleasure "my membership." The next meeting recorded "my resignation." Beside that note there was an asterisk. It read: "required to resign by government decree." One of the conventions of the office of the governor general is a monk-like abstinence from involvement in all external boards and associations.

With this in mind, I proposed to David that if he would remove the asterisk, I would write the foreword. He laughed, and I agreed to his request. I am so glad I did. This book is simply superb. I was completely engrossed and finished it in one sitting. It reinforces three fundamental qualities of David himself: empathy, hope made real, and responsibility.

First, empathy. This is not the same as sympathy—as in, I feel sorry for your fate. Empathy has legs. It means I walk in your shoes. And as I walk with you we come to understand we can do something about fate together.

David was born with empathy genes. He comes from a long line of physicians. While I was at McGill University, when the name Alton Goldbloom was raised, it was almost in a whisper that conveyed respect and awe. He was essentially the father of modern pediatrics there. His legacy lives on decades later in most of the pediatric departments in universities and hospitals across Canada and many in the USA. His two sons were distinguished McGill pediatricians. Richard, David's father, moved to Dalhousie to head pediatrics brilliantly for many years and only retired in his eighties. He and his inimitable wife, Ruth, were the inspiration for so many public good initiatives in Atlantic Canada. It was natural that Richard and Ruth hosted a gathering of the Order of Canada members in Halifax as we conducted a nation-wide consultation on fostering philanthropy and volunteerism in my first year as governor general.

And then came David who took the road less traveled to psychiatry at McGill. He did so because, in his words, there was so much to be done. He was influenced by his father-in-law, a McMaster University psychiatric luminary in the early pioneering days of its innovative medical school.

As I read through these pages, I remembered reading in my teenage days *Dear and Glorious Physician*: a book resonating with empathy about St. Luke recording the stories and parables of Jesus. David begins each chapter with a case of a fictional but entirely believable person and their battle with mental illness. Around that particular story, derived from the thousands of real cases he has seen in his career, he builds a scaffold showing that individual's illness and an innovative approach to diagnosis and care. We, the readers, walk together in that patient's shoes to find a better way forward.

Hope is the second quality. For David, hope is a verb that means to roll up your sleeves. The work he describes is grounded in innovation, doing things better. Minds, like parachutes, work best when open.

These illustrations of innovation, in response to the challenges of mental health, engender pride in our country and how it can do things better. They also resoundingly reaffirm the proposition that curiosity, courage, and collaboration make a difference. The quest for better mental health travels in unprecedented times in Canada. Peter Drucker's observations are applicable: "The greatest danger in turbulent times is not the turbulence. It is to act with yesterday's logic."

That brings us to the third quality: responsibility. David's stories and lessons about the last four decades of mental health emerging from the shadows respond to the challenges of Rabbi Hillel's questions. Asked over two thousand years ago, in modern form they might read, "If not us then who? If not now, then when?"

David's descriptive journey through recent history, the remaking of psychiatry, and a new perspective on mental health bring us to a point of urgency. His trumpet call for action underlines the fact that every year one in five of us will have a serious mental health concern. It is also a challenge at the community and regional level for a collective voice. From hospitals and health providers to the charitable sector, all are called on to collaborate in scaling up more promising innovations. It opens the curtains on mental health forces in Canada, urging our federation to put aside yesterday's logic and embrace seeing mental illness through a new and clearer window. Ultimately, his call is triumphantly optimistic.

To return to the title, *We Can Do Better*, I recall George Bernard Shaw's words: "Some people see things as they are and ask why. Others dream of things that never were and ask why not."

David is an officer of the Order of Canada, our country's highest honour. Its motto is: "We desire a better country." He lives that motto every day, with authenticity and authority. The authenticity is his deep personal engagement in patient care. The authority comes from his working in and leading some of the collaborative networks that bring mental health innovations to life.

The Right Honourable David Johnston,
28th Governor General of Canada
November 2020

INTRODUCTION

◇◇◇◇

I stroll along La Rambla, the broad avenue in central Barcelona, on a sunny spring day in 2017. I slow my pace along the tree-lined street, giving my mind a chance to wander. It might be the jet lag, but there is something vaguely hallucinogenic about the waves and curves of the city's *modernista* architecture. Every building has its own personality and seems to tell a unique story. I pause outside of a century-old home to peer up at the statues adorning it. One figure with a jaunty moustache holds a large, box-shaped camera, while a statue of a stern woman across from him plays a small gramophone—novelty objects now, but ones that would have been at the forefront of technology when the house was built. Sunlight filters through the trees and onto the pavement around me, and I stand still, basking in its warmth and admiring the way the design opens up the streets and gives passersby the ability to see around the corner.

Being open and peeking around the corner are the exact reasons why I am in this charming city in the first place. I am here to attend the twenty-third annual International Conference on Current Issues and Controversies in Psychiatry. Before I am confined to a windowless conference centre for several days, though, I plan to cram in as much tourism as possible. Today is my final day of exploration, so I pull myself away from the streetscape and run to hop on the nearby city bus.

"Where is the stop for Sagrada Familia?" I ask the bus driver after several minutes of staring out the window. He answers in a rapid volley of Spanish that doesn't seem to include the gesture to get out immediately. I politely repeat the question a couple of times with the same result. Eventually he points to the door, because either we have arrived or he is simply fed up with my pestering.

As I come around the corner, my first impression is complete awe. A grand and unfinished project that has outlived its creator, Antoni Gaudí, the Sagrada Familia has a scope and scale that challenges the imagination. It is massive and fantastical—it has the feel of Disney cartoons where trees come to life in a scary way. My eyes are immediately drawn to the church's towers—ornate stone structures that pierce the sky. *It must have taken such incredible imagination,* I think.

As my gaze falls, I am surprised to see cranes and scaffolding dotting the towers and arches of the church's exterior. The modern technology seems out of place, so I approach a nearby guide.

"Excuse me, but what's the reason for the construction?" I ask.

"The church isn't finished," the guide says. "It was started in 1882, but it won't be complete for another decade."

My thoughts go back to the conference, the reason I find myself in this place. The construction of the Sagrada Familia has had to adapt to the rapidly changing urban environment that surrounds the church. Its construction was started at a time when horses were still the primary means of transportation; now a high-speed train runs underneath it. Everything about the church—the lofty ideals that inspired it, the ongoing construction, the mix of old material and new insight—reminds me of our incomplete understanding of and care for people with mental illness. If the church is completed in the twenty-first century, it will be the culmination of two centuries of progress, not all of it smooth. In much the same way, mental health science and treatment have been both controversial and evolving, and the construction is still under way.

The truth is that controversies exist throughout medicine, from the overuse of antibiotics to the value of arthroscopic knee surgery. It is not always easy to find the sweet spot between dealing with uncertainty in medicine and providing hope and reassurance to people who need it. But it's vital that we try.

To my mind, controversy is, to quote Martha Stewart, "a good thing." After all, who would want to work in a field where everything is known and agreed upon? It would bore me beyond belief. But more important, where there is controversy, there is room to learn and improve. That said, few other areas of medicine are as shrouded in uncertainty as psychiatry—from what causes mental illness to what are the most effective treatments—or as mired in controversy about diagnosis, its role in society, and even its theoretical underpinnings.

Physicians (psychiatrists, family doctors, and specialists) and other mental health professionals (psychologists, social workers, occupational therapists, nurses, and other counsellors) disagree on many of those things. But there's one fact on which we all agree: people are suffering. People with mental illnesses, their families and friends, and society at large are all touched by a set of disorders that affect one in five people globally. What is also evident—to every worried parent or partner, to every citizen strolling down a busy downtown street, to every guard working in a prison, to every teacher spending the majority of children's weekday waking hours with them—is that the status quo is unacceptable.

I came of age as a psychiatrist in 1985, when the field was in a state of major change. A seismic shift had occurred when psychiatry turned its back on its heritage of psychoanalysis (still today the popular public perception of the discipline). As psychiatry made its somewhat delayed entry into the mainstream of scientific medicine, it was finally abandoning the long-held views of the origins of mental illnesses—namely, that they could be primarily attributed to early childhood experience and faulty parenting. It was becoming increasingly clear that those traditionally endorsed views could no longer be propped up—we needed a new paradigm. That change wasn't just a matter of updating a textbook or changing a few labels, though. A new direction meant new medical standards; psychiatry had to create an entirely new common language to talk about mental illness. And that, in turn, demanded novel tools and systems to diagnose and treat those illnesses.

At the same time, another insurgency was afoot: the neuroscience revolution was in full flower. Breakthroughs in imaging technology were giving us an unprecedented window onto the brain's structure and function, more refined measures of brain chemistry were allowing us to develop new theories of illness, and genetics was helping us identify vulnerability and risk in new ways.

I was eager to be swept up by and to be a part of this change. When someone has achy joints, headache, sneezing, and a cough, there is a difference between diagnosing the flu based on those symptoms and diagnosing pneumonia based on a chest x-ray and a saliva test. Either illness could fit the symptoms, but better diagnostic tools can paint a deeper, clearer picture. As a young psychiatrist, the breakthroughs in neuroscience and psychiatric practice excited me no end. We were going to be able to help patients better than ever before. Who knew what the future might look like?

I hoped brain imaging might provide an answer. As CAT scans and, later, magnetic resonance imaging became more available technologies—despite the usual Canadian waiting lists—I was eager to order these for patients experiencing their first episode of illness. But no mysteries were ever decoded to guide my understanding or treatment. Although these investigations sometimes provided reassurance to myself and others that I wasn't "missing something" in terms of a nonpsychiatric cause of symptoms, it also inadvertently reinforced for some families the idea that these illnesses weren't "real" because they could not be medically visualized. At the same time, these families knew all too well every pixel of the image of pain and struggle that their son or sister was experiencing. No blood test, whether looking for a faulty thyroid gland or a low vitamin B_{12} level, triggered the "Aha!" moment of Sherlock Holmesian mystery solving. Nevertheless, the tests were dutifully done as part of thoroughness and reassurance of no stone unturned.

By the end of the twentieth century, psychiatry remained virtually alone among the specialties in medicine in its exclusive reliance on clinical symptoms, both observed by physicians and reported by patients, to make diagnoses, to classify disorders, and to guide treatment. Blood tests and brain images were of no help.

Further, the neuroscience revolution did not deliver new treatment tools. Interventions like electroconvulsive therapy, lithium, antidepressants, antipsychotics, and anti-anxiety medications were all available before 1970. While new drugs came along, they generally did not outperform the ones that preceded them but rather offered more therapeutic options and different side effects. And while psychotherapies became briefer in terms of numbers of sessions, more standardized in terms of the actual interventions, and more supported by research evidence, there was no sudden emergence of dramatic superiority of one type over another.

At the same time, progress has been made in medicine more broadly. It has been argued that some of the marked reduction in death rates after heart attack has come not so much from the development of new treatments but rather from the standardization of treatments that we know make a difference. In parallel with neuroscience inquiry into basic underpinnings of mental illness, there has been a significant evolution in developing algorithms and clinical care pathways to guide physicians and patients toward the best evidence-based approaches. While it doesn't eliminate the trial-and-error approach that permeates much of clinical medicine, it does provide physicians with a rationale for the trial sequence based on something more substantial than "the last guy I saw got better with this treatment, so I think I'll try it again" or "the drug rep who came by with doughnuts for my staff said this new pill is really good." Another important element has been measuring change. When we try to quantify the impact of our treatment, it leads to better outcomes because our treatment decisions are not guided by hunches or vague impressions.

Recently, I saw a patient who has struggled for years with a severe depression, at times requiring electroconvulsive therapy. He routinely completes rating scales related to details of his mood. Like many people when they recover from illness, details of his suffering can be mercifully fuzzy for him afterward. His rating-scale score for depression one particular day was low—and well within the range of a healthy, normal mood. He was able to look at his previous scores, and the items he had endorsed, as a way of understanding both how he had once been and the journey he had made. A paper-and-pen test is not expensive technology but rather a ready example of an approach to measurement that can improve care (research indicates that treatment of depression that is data-driven results in better outcomes) as well as patient participation and understanding.

Now, as I approach the latter phase of my career, my sense of the terra incognita of mental health care is even more acute, in terms of both the limits to our understanding and the obstacles to providing better care to more people in need. To put it simply: The status quo is unacceptable. We need to explore new ways of doing things, new routes to people feeling and functioning better. We have good but not great treatments. We have major challenges in accessing help for people who need it. We are nowhere near where we need to be in understanding the brain, the mind, and the interaction of both of them with the environment in ways that would allow us to better predict, prevent, diagnose, and treat. We are beyond choosing between nature and nurture, as we understand increasingly things like how genes can drive our behaviour and how life events and experience can shape our brains. As mental health awareness continues to go up—as it has dramatically in Canada in the last decade—and as stigma recedes, people will rightly expect more and better of mental health care.

For one thing remains constant: people and their experiences of mental illnesses. While clinicians and academics continue to argue over how exactly to use new tools, and quasi-religious schools of psychiatric thought battle for supremacy, people struggling with symptoms continue their journeys, looking for help and for hope.

For me, the core of my work as a psychiatrist has always been trying to understand and help patients and their families. Whether I am acting as a clinician, a teacher, a researcher, an administrator, or an advocate, that has been and always will be the goal. And as much as the first thirty-five years of my career have been rewarding and exciting, I'm still craning my neck around the corner to try to see what could make things better for the people my colleagues and I serve.

What follows is a journey through possibilities. In each chapter, I describe a typical (if there is such a thing when you look closely) case of someone suffering a particular, common illness, although each case is a composite of thousands of patients seen over my career. Each person serves as a springboard for a dive into a new pool of knowledge and treatment. I have purposely not explored those exciting areas of research that may bear fruit in a generation; instead, I have sought out the low-hanging fruit of approaches and models that could make a difference in the lives of patients and families, if accessible to everyone, in the next three to five years. That's a short timeline for innovation. It has been estimated that the lag from scientific discovery to clinical implementation can be as long as seventeen years. But if you are suffering, even three years is a terribly long time to wait.

This journey through innovation isn't meant to be comprehensive. The ideas in these pages are selective rather than exhaustive (and I hope not exhausting)—enticing trailers of brilliant coming attractions that I'm privileged to know about. Over the course of a long career, I have been lucky to meet researchers and clinicians doing exciting work, and so the examples here often come from friends and colleagues from all over the world. Mostly though, I've selected these innovations because together they point to what mental health care could look like if we only embraced such new initiatives.

Some of the pessimism I hear from people about mental illness comes from personal experience, from deep-seated stigma, and from fear of the threat that such illness represents to our uniqueness and identity. And some of it comes from the real failure of existing treatments to meet our high and at times desperate hopes, even though the success rate of most psychiatric treatments is equivalent to that of most medical treatments.

I began writing this book before a coronavirus transformed our world with the COVID-19 pandemic. As I write this paragraph, I am sitting at home instead of at the hospital where I work, seeing patients via secure televideo link rather than in person, maintaining physical distance while finding new ways to connect. While I am glad that people are talking more about the mental health impact of the pandemic on both people who are ill and people providing care for them, the limitation to the help that currently exists also gets highlighted. We are rightly worried about shortages of ventilators, masks, gloves, gowns, and COVID-19 diagnostic tests. But shortages of effective mental health care also need to be addressed as we cope with the impact of the pandemic and its aftermath.

It is a reflection of the growing public awareness of mental health that everyone in Canada, from political leaders to frontline workers in grocery stores and hospitals, is talking about it in the context of the pandemic. At the beginning of May 2020, Prime Minister Justin Trudeau announced a virtual mental health care tool for all Canadians and a commitment of $240 million to support it. A national online portal,

Wellness Together Canada, was quickly created. It offers free of charge wellness self-assessment and tracking, self-guided resources and apps, group coaching and a community of support, and counselling by text or phone. It includes immediate linkage via text to crisis resources for youth, adults, and frontline workers. And it represents a coming together of government, community agencies, and the private sector in common cause to respond to an unprecedented national emergency. Change can happen quickly—within a couple of months of the pandemic disrupting the lives of all Canadians. But what happens when the heat of the crisis inevitably subsides? And what is the impact of COVID-19 on our mental health?

The first hints came from reports of medical workers in Wuhan, China, in February 2020 in terms of overwork, inadequate protection and fear of infection, lack of contact with families, and discrimination, resulting in stress, anxiety, and depression. By late January, guidelines for psychological crisis intervention in the context of the local outbreak had been developed. By March, a review of the evidence of the psychological impact of quarantine and how to reduce it appeared in a major medical journal, again pointing to greater awareness of the mental health impact of a pandemic. At the same time, this is about protecting the mental health of the general population, not that of people who are struggling with a mental illness, and so the solutions are generic and do not medicalize the problem.

Within two months of the onset of the pandemic in Canada, pollsters generated a snapshot of our national mental health through a survey of almost two thousand Canadians. Almost half felt worried or anxious, only 6 percent felt happy, but one-third felt grateful, which may speak to a quality that can help us ride out tough times. Half of Canadians felt COVID had worsened their mental health. That doesn't mean half of Canadians have become mentally ill. In other words, it is actually normal to feel not normal.

But we cannot lose sight, now or later, of the one in five Canadians with mental illness before the pandemic. The pandemic's restrictions on "business as usual" incentivize us to come up with new ways of addressing old problems; it is a helpful accelerant in that regard. And we need to be vigilant about the impact of the pandemic on suicide rates; at least one group has identified the risk as "a perfect storm" with regard to the factors that may increase suicide rates: economic stress, social isolation, decreased access to community and religious support and medical care, worsening of physical illness, and increased firearm sales. At the same time, shared experience and digital community may help to combat these forces.

In July 2020, the human resources firm Morneau Shepell issued its mental health index, which showed a significant decline for Canadians, with financial risk and social isolation driving it downward. In August 2020, the accounting firm Deloitte released its modeling report on the potential impact of COVID on mental health, based on modeling from previous crises and disasters. It predicts a profound impact through economic downturn, with particular impact on women when it comes to employment, income status, and mental health. Finally, a survey released in August 2020 by the US-based Commonwealth Fund, comparing the United States with a number of countries including Canada, shows Americans to be the most vulnerable with regard to lack of access to mental health care, negative economic consequences, and confidence in their government's pandemic response.

COVID has fueled public expectations for faster and better results. Countries are sprinting to vaccine finish lines in months instead of a drug development process that historically was a marathon of many years. Televideo health services have supplanted office and clinic visits. Everything we took for granted about work, school, and social interaction has been challenged. Shaking hands with friends and hugging families now seems so 2019. The need for transformation is urgent, the opportunity is fertile, and the people in need are eager.

What comes next? What needs to change? Are there things already out there that are making a difference beyond our current standards of understanding and care? What holds hope for the future? I'm enough of an optimist—an admittedly incurable one—to believe things can and will be better. We can make a better future. The question is: What will it take?

1

⬦⬦⬦⬦⬦

PIERRE AND ATTENTION DEFICIT HYPERACTIVITY DISORDER

REMOTE COACHING

◇◇◇◇

Hold the Phone

Pierre was a rambunctious young boy, always in motion—a "whirling dervish," his mother, Eloise, called him. His father, Stephane, recognized himself in Pierre, both with pride and a little bit of dread as he anticipated what school would be like for his son.

By the time Pierre was in grade one, what had seemed like relentless curiosity and exuberance began to clash with rules, schedules, and even learning. He struggled to stay seated in the classroom or to wait his turn when the teacher asked a question. Instead, he often disrupted the class with blurted jokes and laughter, physical restlessness, and a tendency to take things from other children. It meant frequent trips to the hallway and twice to the principal's office. At times, as the teacher spoke to the students, Pierre seemed a million miles away, staring out the window, seemingly transfixed by a squirrel on a tree branch. When the children were asked to bring something from home for show-and-tell, Pierre frequently forgot or misplaced his items, and he tuned out when reprimanded about it.

Pierre's teacher and his parents were worried about his ability to succeed in school and to make friends. Keeping him busy was helpful, but it didn't always translate into keeping him engaged. The teacher suggested that Pierre's family doctor be involved and that the parents complete one of the common questionnaires used to consider the possibility of attention deficit/hyperactivity disorder (ADHD). "That's what they said I had," noted his father, "and so did two of my brothers. They put us all on Ritalin. My parents said it helped."

Stephane felt guilty that he had passed on to his son a vulnerability to a disorder that wreaked some havoc on Stephane's own childhood. Like many people with ADHD, Stephane had outgrown the symptoms as an adult—but he had never forgotten them. He suddenly had a new appreciation for his own parents' struggles in raising him.

The family doctor asked Pierre's parents and teacher to complete a brief survey. They reviewed the results and noticed the overwhelming number of boxes ticked under the "very much" column describing ADHD symptoms. The doctor decided to prescribe Ritalin for Pierre and encouraged his parents to visit some ADHD websites for further information and support. "I'm afraid that's all I can do," she said.

Pierre took Ritalin and the effects were evident both at home and in the classroom within a couple of weeks. Pierre seemed calmer, more able to focus and sit still. He wasn't sent to the hallway anymore for being disruptive and seemed to enjoy being part of the class more. His symptoms were certainly better, but they weren't gone, and Eloise and Stephane felt that their son needed more than pills could provide. They wanted strategies that would help them cope better as a family, as well as skills that Pierre could use in situations that brought out the worst of his diagnosis.

But getting in to see the school psychologist or a child psychiatrist would take many months, and seeing a psychologist in private practice was beyond their means. It was hard enough for them to coordinate taking time away from their jobs in the middle of a weekday to meet with the teacher, let alone ongoing sessions with a counsellor.

◇◇◇◇

ADHD, sometimes shortened to ADD, is one of those sets of initials that people now use casually in everyday conversation as a kind of short-hand—"I'm so ADD today I can't find my car keys." It's much the same with how people refer to obsessive-compulsive disorder (OCD)—"I like to keep my DVDs organized by movie genre; I know it's so OCD of me." Some could argue that this represents greater literacy or acceptance of mental illness, but I don't buy it. To me, it is a trivialization of illness, a self-mocking joke that betrays a lack of awareness of just how debilitating, intrusive, and persistent the symptoms can be.

That being said, ADHD is more recognized, diagnosed, and treated than ever before, especially in adults. While some children outgrow ADHD symptoms, long-term follow-up studies show that symptoms can persist into adulthood. For adults I see who are questioning whether this explains their difficulties, the answer is: sometimes but not always. In adults, there is often a clear history of ADHD symptoms persisting since childhood, corroborated by parents and old report cards. For those adults whose symptoms developed only in their thirties, in my experience it is far more likely that their concentration and focus difficulties are aspects of a depression or anxiety disorder—or sometimes a profound dislike of the task that requires their attention.

According to the Canadian ADHD Resource Alliance (CADDRA) 2018 treatment guidelines, clinical descriptions of the behaviour patterns go back to the late 1700s and the benefits of amphetamine drugs for the symptoms were first observed in the late 1930s. So this is not simply a recent fad, despite growing recognition and treatment.

In 2014, a careful review of the previous three decades found no increase in how commonly ADHD occurred among children in community samples. This is opposed to the rise in the number of children being given the diagnosis by health professionals, which, according to the US National Institutes of Health, increased between 2003 and 2011 by 42 percent. That's a total increase from 8 percent to 11 percent of all children.

This is a cause for concern for many: from parents to policy makers, philosophers to health care providers, ethicists to educators. People worry about overdiagnosis and overtreatment. However, few people argue that ADHD doesn't exist. So where is the sweet spot between missing cases and overcalling them?

In Canada, while the number of cases of ADHD increased significantly between 1999 and 2012, most of the diagnoses were made by family physicians. Diagnoses of ADHD were made in 3 to 5 out of every 100 children and youth, with significant variability across provinces. And it is estimated that when the diagnosis is made, stimulant medication follows in the majority of cases.

Without a diagnostic blood or imaging test, ADHD remains a clinical diagnosis, often supported by multi-perspective questionnaires completed by teachers, parents, and the people who may have the disorder. The consequences of missing the diagnosis can include a very negative impact on school performance and in developing a social network—the principal jobs of children. On the other hand, overdiagnosis can lead to labeling that may be stigmatizing, treatment that may not be necessary or helpful, and a blind eye to other factors contributing to the way the child is functioning.

Not every person who clicks his ballpoint pen repeatedly, shifts in his chair, or tunes out has ADHD, in the same way that not everyone who burps has acid reflux and not everyone with chest pain has heart disease. But a recognizable pattern of co-occurring symptoms that are both sustained and having a negative impact on school and social performance are at the heart of the diagnosis of ADHD.

I have to admit that in the first half of my career I never used to think about this diagnosis as an adult psychiatrist. I had seen children with ADHD during my child psychiatry training but hadn't been sufficiently curious to wonder what happens to them when they grow up.

In my own dim way, I wrongly saw age eighteen as some kind transformation point and didn't ask adults about ADHD symp as public awareness has grown and online self-assessments pr Dr. Google have proliferated, more adults are wondering wh explains how they think and function.

That being said, the primary province of ADHD, where likely to emerge and play havoc, is childhood. That's where m help is needed.

Given how long it will take for Pierre to see a school psych a child psychiatrist outside of the school system, it is easy to ass simply having more such mental health experts available will problem. That isn't the case, though. We know from studies of trist supply conducted in Ontario that the problem of accessing isn't any better in regions with higher concentrations of these sp such as major urban centres, than it is in rural areas. And it's n the case that people need the level of expertise of those profess not everyone with a headache needs to see a neurologist and n one with high blood pressure needs to see a cardiologist. The r mismatch between problems and solutions.

We will never have—nor should we—enough child psychi see every young person with mental health problems and illness though we could make better use of a larger contingent of them. need is a greater range of services for young people of differing intensity and expertise so we can match level of need with approp sources, including the most advanced and specialized, at the right fact, that's what we need throughout our entire mental health care

There is an old *New Yorker* cartoon of someone flailing i and, on seeing a faithful collie barking on the banks of the river to her, "Lassie, get help!" In the next frame of the cartoon, Lass her back on a chaise longue, speaking to a therapist. Funny? Sure me, it says we need to broaden our reality as well as our popular conception of what getting help means.

Even if a greater number of psychiatrists would improve access for people like Pierre, it wouldn't happen overnight. It can take up to fifteen years of postsecondary education and training to launch a child psychiatrist. It's not just a question of improving access to existing resources but also of connecting people with appropriate new resources. There are opportunities to diversify the mental health workforce, training up much more quickly people who can deliver evidence-based treatments that can effectively meet people's needs. It means shaking up how we think about care and care providers. It means leveraging existing knowledge of innovative approaches that work. Innovation is what Pierre needs, as long as it is supported by credible evidence that the approach makes a positive difference. Oxford University Press publishes a series of books called Treatments That Work—a sobering reminder that not everything we think of as treatment has evidence to support its benefits.

Not only are wait lists long, and the costs of ongoing treatment too high for many families, but traditional services are typically available during weekday business hours, often when families have the least flexibility to get together. Children should spend their days in school; it is their ticket to chances for a better life—and better mental health—as an adult. And parents are often themselves busy with work commitments, where taking time off for appointments can be a significant challenge. Mental illnesses like ADHD can be a real barrier to the success of children and families, and so we need alternative approaches.

For Pierre's family and so many like them, there is a need for available, affordable, accessible, evidence-based services beyond the traditional format of office- or institution-based weekday clinical practices. What many Canadian parents like Eloise and Stephane don't know is that some of these innovative resources already exist. One such program has incredible potential to provide help for families like theirs: the Strongest Families Institute (SFI).

SFI is the brainchild of Patrick McGrath, an academic and clinical psychologist, and Patricia "Trish" Lingley-Pottie, a PhD nurse in Halifax,

Nova Scotia. The origins of SFI go back forty years to when Patrick was in Ottawa dealing with children who suffered from chronic pain. He developed a technique of using coaches to help kids and their families via telephone—an early form of e-health long before smartphones, apps, and the internet. It was an academic success but an innovation failure because there was no significant uptake. Canada is sometimes called the land of pilot projects, where great ideas are generated and validated but not scaled up—whether due to lack of political will, funding, technology, or vision to transform the local to the national.

Nevertheless, Patrick knew that many people lived far away from specialized treatment resources or could not meet the demands of daytime weekday appointments that disrupted school for the child and work for the parents. And many more children struggle with emotional and behavioural problems than with chronic pain. So he shifted his clinical focus from pain to mental health, and not long after, SFI was born.

The goal of SFI, and similar programs that would follow, is to help children with symptoms of ADHD, disruptive behaviour, anxiety disorder, and persistent bedwetting by teaching them, and their families, strategies and skills for dealing with specific situations, thoughts, and feelings that triggered their symptoms. When he designed the program, Patrick carefully reviewed the scientific evidence to support those strategies and created manuals that specially trained coaches could use when speaking with families over the phone.

Coaches encourage parents to pay heed to the times when their child is being attentive, making sure positive behaviours at home and in school are reinforced through reward systems. They can help parents break down tasks into specific, manageable goals. And they can teach parents how to use problem-solving strategies that include the child in the plan, that help the child with focus and emotion regulation. The manuals were effectively scripts, and they included prompts to remind the coaches to use role-playing and problem-solving skills with children and parents. The program also provided handbooks for children and parents and complementary audio and video products that demonstrate the skills in action.

Each session between the coach and the family is conducted over the phone. It starts with a conversation in which the coach uses a series of screening tools to identify what the problem areas are and, more important, how to help deal with them. To minimize bias, screening is done by a separate department—evaluation assistants—using validated scales such as the Brief Child and Family Phone Interview (developed by academics at McMaster University more than a decade ago) and the Strengths and Difficulties Questionnaire (well established internationally as a screening tool). All the resulting data is entered into a care plan page and a problem identification dashboard on a computer program that families can access.

The telephone sessions are held in the evenings, when families are most often available—there are no office visits, no travel, and no delays. Of course, in the context of pandemic isolation (as of this writing), families have become even more available together. Coaches also aim to deliver written results in ways that families will understand, preferring short, graphic-heavy reports over lengthy narratives that too often cause patients' eyes to glaze over.

It's important to recognize that SFI does not make formal diagnoses, even though it focuses on clinical problems; in most jurisdictions, providing a formal diagnosis is restricted to physicians and psychologists. But you don't need an MD or a PhD to spot a problem, and sometimes referral to SFI follows a more formal diagnostic evaluation by a health professional. In essence, SFI is focused on addressing symptoms. And that matches up well with what people want from mental health care in general; people are more distressed by specific symptoms than by the labels that categorize them. Symptoms are what people have, while diagnoses are what professionals make.

SFI goes right to the heart of that, teaching skills for handling those symptoms. The process helps parents learn to deal with a range of common childhood behaviour problems, such as temper outbursts, not listening, verbal and physical aggression, and difficulties with focus—common struggles in children with ADHD. The calls aren't long—typically only forty-five minutes, once a week. And despite the availability of newer forms of communication like FaceTime, Zoom, or Skype, SFI still advocates for the use of telephones. They found that many families didn't want to "see" their coach, and the visual anonymity of the phone meant that families often disclosed more. They liken it to the confessional screen of the Catholic Church, and it serves as a reminder that while we are easily attracted by the shiniest technology, it is the substance of what is transmitted that counts more than the vehicle for it.

When I listened to a forty-five-minute phone call used in training between a parent and a coach, I did so as a mental health professional and a parent. I was impressed from both perspectives. The call began with a review of progress since the previous call, and it felt natural and conversational, not a lecture or a scripted dialogue. It was very much rooted in the realities of that particular child and family, both supporting and challenging the parent to consider alternative ways of responding to their child and to reflect on the consequences of rewarding behaviour, bad and good. At one point, the coach role-played the child to get the parent to demonstrate her responses and then consider their impact. At another time, the coach and parent listened to an audio recording of an interaction in order both to appraise how it went and to imagine alternate responses. Throughout, the coach was practical, positive, and supportive. There was a palpable relationship, even on the phone, between the coach and the parent. And it wasn't just about exploring what went wrong in the past week; there was also discussion of what went well and why. Seamlessly, rating scales were introduced to evaluate both the progress to date since beginning the program and the value of the previous session.

As a mental health professional, I could feel the coach carefully positioning the health-promoting bricks to create a stronger foundation. I heard cognitive behavioural techniques used alongside positive regard for the child and family—but always in the context of the actual experiences of the people on the other end of the line. It never felt generic, stilted, or forced.

As a parent, admittedly through the gauze of distant memory, I could see things I wish I had done differently, even though I have been blessed with two terrific sons. All children challenge us as parents, and all of us as parents can benefit from strategies such as the ones I heard. One of my favourite child-rearing books from almost seventy years ago, by pediatrician and psychiatrist Dr. Hilde Bruch, had a great title: *Don't Be Afraid of Your Child: A Guide for Perplexed Parents*. I treasure my vintage copy.

But some children and families really need more intensive help, and that's where SFI can be an important first step (and sometimes the only step). As a first step, it's important that it be rapidly accessible. Families are typically contacted within forty-eight hours of receipt of a referral for an initial assessment, and often start treatment within three weeks of that first contact. That's fast.

Because the SFI coaches are nonclinicians, it is much easier and faster to expand this kind of parent training program to reach more people than it is to train up and distribute more child psychologists and psychiatrists. Coaches tend to be women in their mid-twenties who are experienced in working with children and families in some way, usually with an undergraduate degree as well as some customer-service experience or a background as a personal support worker or a teacher. There are long-standing male staff as well, but regardless of gender, coaches are typically people drawn toward caring and nurturing services. And that's what I heard on the training call—an empathic, supportive, and encouraging voice of a person who seemed very skilled in promoting self-reflection, consideration of alternative approaches, and engagement in change exercises. Although it is manual-driven, the casual and conversational nature of the interaction conceals its theoretical under-pinnings and prescribed interventions.

The training is intensive, and within two weeks most coaches are starting with closely supervised cases. A month into the job, coaches are carrying a full caseload of thirty people. Most of them work full-time in that capacity.

That ability to quickly ramp up the readiness of coaches is a strik-ing contrast to traditional health care training, which takes place over a number of years. More and more across the field of mental health, organizations are discovering that they can provide new levels of service by rapidly deploying people with less training than traditional health care professionals. That less intensive training is balanced by the coach's willingness to be monitored, supervised, and taught by experts. Indeed, in the experience of the creators of SFI, who have also worked in tra-ditional health care settings, most coaches are more open to auditing, evaluation, and feedback than are seasoned health professionals.

As a psychiatrist, it is rare for my work to be closely scrutinized by my colleagues or my superiors, unless there has been a complaint filed or a concern voiced. That makes it difficult to ensure quality control beyond my initial formal training (which ended thirty-five years ago, although fortunately my patients kept teaching me long after my super-visors gave up). Like many professionals, I earn continuing education credits by attending courses and lectures to keep my skills and knowl-edge current, but that is not the same. Beyond the lack of accountabil-ity, I also think the secrecy that surrounds some mental health clinical work, while providing assurance around confidentiality, also contrib-utes to a sense of mystery and uncertainty about what clinicians actually do. In SFI, coaches are expected to "show their work" just as we all had to do in math class.

The flexibility of the SFI model applies not just to how the coaches train, but also how and when they work. SFI coaches typically work out of a call centre, but they can operate from any secure location as long as certain privacy standards are met. They're also prepared to work evenings and nights, when parents are most available, which is different from the vast majority of traditional mental health professionals.

Historically, child and youth mental health services have been publicly criticized for long waiting lists to see highly specialized clinicians. While in Canada we are accustomed to waiting months and even years for some non-emergency procedures for adults (think eyes, hips, and knees), similar waiting lists for children are indefensible. Consider how few years they have been alive and how critical an intervention can be to their growth and success. When the existing complement of clinicians is limited in relation to the needs of the population, it's not feasible to ask them to work longer hours to meet demand; they are already working very hard. And simply increasing the number of them is a solution that will take years of training to materialize. Rather, we need to think pragmatically about different and new resources that can be marshalled to provide evidence-based help more quickly. If they can only target people with mild to moderate symptoms, then those who are more severely affected can still use more intensive and specialized existing services.

Families need to be and to feel part of the solution throughout the life span, but nowhere more so than in the lives of children and youth. I remember when my father, Richard Goldbloom, the former pediatrician-in-chief at the Izaak Walton Killam Hospital for Children in Nova Scotia, set up a pioneering "Care by Parent" inpatient unit at the hospital, where parents were expected to stay overnight with their children and be active participants in treatment. Some more traditional clinicians viewed this as an intrusion at the time. They changed their tune when they experienced its value in clinical care. And my late father-in-law, Nathan Epstein, former chair of psychiatry at McMaster and Brown universities, devoted his clinical and academic career to understanding and treating families. So I have a bias: We mental health professionals need to view families as both experts and collaborators. SFI tries to harness the power of families to make change happen during the many hours and days between sessions.

In SFI programs for children twelve and under, dealing with behaviour difficulties, anxiety, and nighttime bedwetting engages the whole family. Bedwetting is common and normal before the age of five, until children increasingly gain control of their bladders. But after that, it can both create problems (shame, barriers to socializing with friends through sleepovers, etc.) and reflect problems (including problems in adapting to changes like a new home, a new sibling, etc.). In children ages five to twelve, when there is no history of dry periods at night and bedwetting persists, this is called primary enuresis. It is here that an SFI intervention can make a difference. If bedwetting starts after a sustained period of dry nights, that is called secondary enuresis and may require a different approach to understanding and treatment than what SFI offers. It may need more traditional evaluation for the emotional, physical, and environmental factors that have triggered a return to bedwetting.

For primary enuresis, SFI combines urine-sensitive alarms with positive reward systems to motivate children to be dry at night. When helping children and youth aged thirteen and up, there is less parent involvement. That being said, the parents still have a role, and there are resources for them, including tips from the SFI's web-based software on how to handle their child.

This software is called IRIS—Intelligent Research and Intervention Software. The same way that the iris is the structure in the eye that determines how much light reaches the human retina, so does IRIS help illuminate solutions to problems that arise from behavioural challenges. Further, it takes information specific to clients—ages, interests—and weaves it into suggestions and recommendations, making them all the more "personal." Trish Lingley-Pottie refers to IRIS as "she," reflecting our relentless need to humanize machines—and because it happens to be a female first name.

IRIS begins collecting data as soon as the referral is made to SFI, either with staff entering demographic information from a paper referral or with families entering personal details through the secure SFI portal. She has a sophisticated artificial intelligence and learns quickly (unlike me). Her design includes sending parents a series of alerts, tasks, steps, and timelines. If parents are uncomfortable with this online interaction, IRIS can interact with their coach.

Based on the information parents provide, IRIS customizes and contextualizes its exercises and examples so it "fits" that particular child and family. For instance, if a three-year-old child likes to play with blocks (I still do, although I have to share with my grandchildren), IRIS autopopulates all areas within the seventeen sessions of intervention with block-playing examples to teach and reinforce skills. She also provides scoring of measures and creation of dashboards to track progress. She draws on a library of audio examples of interactions between parents and children that demonstrate skills, making sure they are relevant to the child and family. This is a good example of mental health catching up with what online stores and video streaming services have known how to do for some time—to personalize offers and recommendations based on your patterns and preferences. And this is not static; IRIS is continuously learning more about its users and modifying its prompts, examples, and exercises. It is the antithesis of one-size-fits-all.

Families have access to IRIS as soon as they enter the program. They can also enter their outcome evaluations to track progress and shape feedback and intervention. IRIS's algorithm sends automated tips and reminders after each coaching session to promote skill acquisition. That's more than most of us clinicians do between appointments. In other words, between sessions with the coach, the family is engaged through IRIS, and coaching sessions provide observations on progress since the last appointment as well as plans for the future. It is a type of measurement-based care, and there is evidence in psychiatry that when measurement is a standard part of treatment, outcomes improve. This kind of measurement involves using rating scales rather than relying on the general impression of either the patient or the clinician, as in the cryptic progress note in a clinical record that simply says, "Improved." According to who and according to what?

The program isn't streamlined just for patients—it helps ease the burden on coaches and staff, too. In its latest version, IRIS comes with quality assurance algorithms, triggers and flags, an outcome repository of ratings that answer the key question of whether someone got better, and the capacity to generate a range of reports for parents and coaches. It reduces organizational waste, which is no small thing: the less time staff have to devote to managing files, the more they can focus on client care. No one outside SFI has access to the IRIS repositories, but the technology can create aggregated summary reports of multiple users that can be sent to funders—a level of accountability that funders see all too infrequently.

The functionality of IRIS is focused (not to milk the eyeball metaphor too much) on acquiring and reinforcing skills, tracking symptoms, and reporting outcomes. It is personalized and customized to gender, including nonbinary options, and other elements of diversity, such as culture and ethnoracial heritage, can be customized by the coach.

The focus on individual care also means that cultural competency and diversity sensitivity are core values of SFI. Canada's treatment of indigenous peoples—their rights and their health—is a stain on the country's history. The growing awareness of the need to codevelop mental health services in partnerships that reflect the experience and values of individuals and communities is an important theme of twenty-first-century care, one that we need to increasingly build into our health care models. SFI has a long history of involvement with Eskasoni First Nation, the largest indigenous community in Atlantic Canada. And, as we will see in the next chapter, this Mi'kmaq community is also one of the sites for the largest mental health system transformation initiatives in Canada that is focused on youth. Other marginalized communities include people in remote areas, on low income, or with low literacy; they can receive SFI programs that are customized by coaches who are trained in that task. Programs like SFI can help pave the way for not just better health care, but better understanding of the many barriers people face.

This culture of the organization is part of what makes SFI so successful. Although the treatments are standardized and sessions are audited, there is room for individual clinical judgment and customization. Coaches routinely seek input from their supervisors in complex situations, and they are scored on their competency, something that rarely happens with traditional mental health professionals. As I said earlier, in those traditional roles, we professionals are most likely to be scrutinized when there is a complaint about our care, rather than in a systematic, universal, and recurring way.

For SFI coaches, their service is ranked by quality—including client satisfaction—but also quantity; the coaches have benchmarks they need to meet in terms of the number of cases they handle per year, attrition rates (how many people drop out), and the timeliness of their service. No psychiatrist is systematically evaluated in that way, whether they work with children or adults. If a case has shown no progress over two weeks, IRIS flags the situation for the coach's manager. That is a very short time frame for expecting progress, but it holds both coaches and families to a high level of expectation—and no one has ever complained that "I got better too fast."

However, some traditional psychotherapists have viewed rapid recovery, without exploration of deeper "root causes," as a form of avoidance and escape called "flight into health." It's not a compliment on rapid transit. Exploring root causes, though, is something SFI does not do— not that root causes are necessarily knowable. And sometimes people, especially young people, can and do get better quickly. Also, two weeks in the life of children is a bigger chunk of time than for adults. If there is no progress, the flag triggers a review of the file by the supervisor, who will then work with the coach to determine if additional training or role playing with the coach is needed—or if anything else is needed to maximize the likelihood of success. There is a weekly "coaches' corner" (without the colourful jackets or inappropriate remarks seen and heard until recently on hockey broadcasts) for group input and guidance. And if things are getting worse, there is a mechanism for alerting local mental health agencies of the need for a higher-level intervention.

The use of standardized, regular outcome measurement in SFI's programs answers an important question: How do we know a treatment is working for us? It's a critical element of SFI that is too often missing from twentieth- and even some twenty-first-century treatments. It's not enough anymore for a clinician or a coach—or a child or parent— to say, "things seem better to me." Those entirely subjective appraisals can sometimes reflect reality, but they're also affected by bias and hope. Without measurement, we can be blind to lack of progress in a person's condition or even worsening of it. As I've already noted, there is already good scientific evidence that when we measure progress, it leads to better outcomes. But it also creates a shared language and partnership between the person providing care and the person receiving it.

Otherwise, people may not be on the same page as to what constitutes a good outcome. When I was a medical intern late in the last century, we used to talk about patients who "died with good electrolytes"—that we had done a really excellent job of making sure that their sodium and potassium levels were normal, but unfortunately they succumbed to their illness. It was glib, gallows humour in a context where we were exposed to death at close range more regularly than most young people in their careers. But it is also a reminder to consider the relevance of what is being measured. A quotation often attributed to Albert Einstein, but which may be from the sociologist William Cameron, bears repeating: "Not everything that can be counted counts, and not everything that counts can be counted."

The other important element of SFI—the use of interventions that have a foundation in evidence—answers an even broader question: How do I know this treatment works for most people? This revolves around the intersection between the power of science and the hunger of hope. Desperation can lead people down blind alleys of treatments that promise help but have no data to prove that they deliver. For children living with ADHD, like Pierre, naturopathic remedies and restrictive diets are readily available as treatments—but the scientific evidence that they work is much harder to find. By moving toward programs that follow and further develop the SFI model, we will be able to prove what treatments work and who they help—something we desperately need. We already have good data on traditional treatments like stimulants for ADHD based on decades of research.

SFI was initially met with skepticism, but its emphasis on data, benchmarks, and outcomes convinced the government in Nova Scotia it was a worthwhile investment. The program was also viewed with some fear that it would take people away from traditional treatment resources, even though those resources already had enormous wait lists. Fear of change and protection of turf can generate resistance, even when existing treatments are not meeting demand or are not providing the evidence that supports their value. Fortunately, the skepticism and the fear quickly subsided, and SFI has reduced those wait lists dramatically. More than that, mainstream clinicians were soon happy to have SFI as a frontline resource to which they could refer patients rather than have them sit on waiting lists.

Programs like SFI are great examples of the new ways that people can receive help for common mental health problems and illnesses. For some people, like Pierre and his family, it will be all they need. They may learn enough skills and strategies, rapidly and in a convenient way, to cope with his ADHD so that both he and his parents feel and function better, even if he ultimately also needs medication. For others, it will be the first step in a journey that progresses to more specialized treatment. But in a mental health care system with limited and stretched resources, the goal should be to find the least intrusive, least intensive treatment that makes a meaningful, measurable difference to someone's symptoms, problems, functioning, and quality of life.

Currently, there is little logic in who gets what kind of help; it can be more a reflection of where you live, how much money you have, or who you know. Some people end up getting no help at all, while others use highly specialized resources when a simpler intervention could work. In fact, this isn't just an issue for mental health care; it's about how we approach health in general.

For those with access to resources and means, frequent "complete check-ups"—blood tests, imaging studies, consultation with specialists, etc.—trump logic and clinical need, and don't lead to better results. My father, a pediatrician and a believer in innovation and evidence, often likes to define a healthy person as someone who hasn't been adequately investigated. He's also, of course, a wag, but his point is a good one.

The alternative is called a stepped-care approach. Imagine a pyramid. People with the mildest difficulties are at the bottom, receiving the least intensive and least specialized care. The most complex individuals and situations make up the top of the pyramid, where the most expert and specialized resources are gathered. This makes more sense than one-size-fits-all or first-come, first-served models that result in mismatches between needs and treatments.

SFI was envisioned as a way of helping people with mild-to-moderate difficulties, leaving the more severe cases to traditional routes and expertise. Patrick and Trish envisioned SFI as a first step in a stepped-care model, a program to which a teacher or health professional might refer someone after minimal screening to ensure the person does not immediately need more intensive services. However, SFI is proving to be of help to families whose difficulties traverse the full range of severity.

SFI has yet to be rolled out fully across Canada, but it is growing. In 2010, it was successfully exported to Calgary, then Edmonton and rural Alberta. It also exists as a bilingual service in the four Atlantic provinces, in several parts of Ontario, and for all military and veterans' families across the country. It has been recognized for its breakthroughs, most recently receiving the Governor General's Award for Innovation in 2017 and, prior to that, similar awards from the Mental Health Commission of Canada and the Ernest C. Manning Foundation. In 2018, five thousand children and youth and their families in Canada were involved with SFI interventions. It's even been adopted internationally, with Finland, Vietnam, and New Zealand introducing the service in some form. The CEO of SFI reported in 2019 that successful outcomes of treatment are as high as 91 percent, with a dropout rate of only 6 percent. And the outcomes do not vary significantly by community—be they urban, rural, remote, or indigenous.

In an ideal world, then, this type of care should be available to anyone. So why isn't it? There are two major obstacles to scaling it up: money, and ensuring that the right leadership is in place to oversee rapid expansion. The question of money is for politicians and policy advisors to address. As for leadership, coaches can be trained rapidly, but maintaining a consistent quality of service and outcomes requires experienced supervisors and maintaining proven standards. It takes up to two years to gain the experience to be a fully effective supervisor, and because the nature of SFI requires evening work, so that it fits to the schedules of families, it can be a challenge to attract people to the role. Still, SFI is growing and moving relentlessly westward across Canada, albeit not fast enough in relation to the need.

In the current model, it costs about $1,000 per family for seventeen fifty-minute weekly sessions over five months—and that includes all the operational costs of running SFI as well as providing sessions, all educational materials used by families, and summary letters at the end. Families can choose to participate in one-on-one coaching or group coaching, where they learn from other families grappling with the same problems as well as from the coach. Funding primarily comes from provincial governments, with some philanthropic matching grants.

Pierre faced multiple obstacles in traditional care: long wait times and further barriers of cost and scheduling. Initiatives like SFI help to overcome these.

It used to be said that two of Nova Scotia's greatest exports were fish and brains. SFI definitely falls into the latter category. SFI has the potential to provide a valuable and proven first step (and, for some, the only step needed) for young people and their families in addressing common and impairing mental health problems like ADHD. It's a cost-effective solution that's having a profound positive impact on families, the sort of sound investment of public and private health care dollars and stepped-care approach that can serve as a model for a new way forward. For children like Pierre and their families, it can mean better management of symptoms and better functioning at school and at home—building blocks for anyone's success.

2

◇◇◇◇◇

SHOBHA AND ANXIETY

INTEGRATED YOUTH SERVICES

◇◇◇◇

Lower the Bar (to Entry)

Shobha didn't know what to do. At age seventeen, she found herself struggling with anxiety, feeling depressed and overwhelmed, and isolated from her small circle of friends. Compounding her struggle was a deep-seated sense of shame that she was in this predicament, as her parents had made a difficult decision to leave extended family and established work in India to make a better life for their children in Canada. Her father, formerly an engineer, was now driving an airport limousine, and her mother, who had been a teacher, was now cleaning office buildings.

Shobha saw how hard they worked without complaining and what they had sacrificed. How could she burden them with her problems? Even though at times she felt so bad she wished she were dead, she knew that within her family and her community mental health problems were not discussed or considered legitimate—unless they were at the extreme of her father's cousin Arjun, who had spent his entire adult life in an asylum and was referred to as "crazy Arjun" as if it were his full name.

Shobha's family doctor provided care for her entire family and sometimes spoke with her parents in Hindi, which Shobha couldn't fully follow. He was older than Shobha's father and she found him patronizing and old-school, and she had little confidence that what she told him wouldn't find its way back to her parents. She couldn't ask him for birth control pills, let alone discuss her emotional state. At school, the counselling office often had a long queue of students against the wall, reminding Shobha of those TV shows where victims try to pick their assailant out of a lineup. So that option was out for her; she felt it would be like painting "Loser" on her sweatshirt.

At the same time, she didn't know what was wrong with her; she didn't use to feel like this. She felt too embarrassed to talk to friends and too afraid to talk to health professionals. She felt, in this moment, particularly alone and uncertain about what to do.

◇◇◇◇

Shobha is facing a familiar dilemma for young people struggling with their mental health. Even though there are resources in the medical system and within her school, availability doesn't equate with access or compatibility. She has a doctor she can't completely relate to or trust with confidential information, she has a school counsellor in a setting where she feels exposed to her peers and possibly judged by them—and even then, the help they can provide comes with a waiting list. She finds it very hard to wait when she doesn't know exactly what's wrong or what she needs. But she does know she feels embarrassed and even worthless at times. And it's not who she used to be.

Our traditional ways of providing help to young people through private office practices, clinics, and hospitals are not meeting needs for access and intervention among young people. Too often, this translates into no treatment, delayed treatment, or use of emergency rooms as points of first contact when untreated illness has worsened in severity. This delay costs young people precious time in terms of lost productivity, functioning, and well-being, and it costs society in terms of care in expensive settings (like emergency rooms). That's not how entry into care should begin.

I'm certainly not the only one who sees this problem. Ashok Malla is a psychiatrist at McGill University and an internationally recognized leader in research and clinical innovation in the area of early intervention with youth. A South Asian man of medium build, his appearance is distinguished by penetrating gray-green eyes, a shaved head, and a calm demeanour that evokes an ancient statue.

Ashok and I first met more than twenty years ago. Even then his focus was on early intervention, but at the time specifically in young people with first-episode psychosis, the term used to describe the initial appearance of an illness like schizophrenia. It often begins in one's late teens and early twenties, with the potential to derail the trajectory of a life, especially if the first episode is followed by more episodes. This meant not only starting treatment sooner but also working differently than the traditional way; treatment was about more than medication alone and was tailored to the life stage needs of young people and their families. Reorganization of clinical services to promote early intervention in first-episode psychosis is one of the evidence-based changes to our mental health system that has been implemented broadly across Canada and internationally. And that type of service delivery change is an enduring and consistent theme in Ashok's work for more than two decades in Ontario and Quebec.

At the beginning of his career in the 1980s, Ashok became aware of two things: the role of stress, even in major illnesses like schizophrenia and bipolar disorder, and the sense that by the time he saw patients, they had been ill for far too long. He recalled taking a walk along the canals in Rotterdam after meeting with colleagues who were doing early intervention work in Australia and Norway and thinking, *We've got to do this.* Indeed, this was his first encounter with Dr. Pat McGorry, an Australian hailed as the godfather of early intervention. Ashok realized that treatment for young people with psychosis needed to occur sooner and be different, with better incorporation of social skills training and family intervention that had proven their value but were not routinely offered. By the mid-1990s, that is exactly what he was doing. While medications played a crucial role in quelling the torment of hearing voices and having terrifying paranoid beliefs, learning skills to navigate the journey to a meaningful and productive life were also crucial. He and others showed that as the duration of untreated illness decreased, outcomes improved. For people whose abilities to interact in a healthy way in relationships or perform at work or in school suffered when they became ill, coaching helped them to get back on track with things that are all too often taken for granted. Families learned skills in communication and interaction as well as knowledge about illness and coping strategies.

He thinks that today, clinicians are very good at providing service to the people who come to see them, but less good at thinking about the people who don't come—and why they aren't seen. That makes sense. As clinicians, our first priority is understandably the person sitting in front of us in our offices and clinics, not the invisible person who hasn't found the right door to enter.

And that was the impetus for perhaps the crowning achievement of his long career: ACCESS Open Minds/Esprits Ouverts (AOM). The AOM project is one of the largest funded health care research projects in Canadian history, focusing on improving the connection between youth and mental health services. It's a multi-province initiative, sponsored by the Canadian Institutes of Health Research and the Graham Boeckh Foundation in Montreal, a private family foundation dedicated to improvement in mental health services. (Full disclosure: I sit on the board of this foundation and serve on the national advisory committee of AOM; however, I joined the board after it began funding this initiative.) While the name ACCESS suggests merely getting people help, it represents much more than that: it actually stands for Adolescent/young adult Connections to Community-driven, Early, Strengths-based and Stigma-free services. You can see why an acronym was needed.

AOM is informed by the science of early case identification and its positive impact on the outcome of treatment. And just as important, it addresses the fact that rates of untreated mental illness in Canada are unacceptably high (while access to treatments is unacceptably low)— and this state of affairs would not be tolerated for any other form of illness. With mental health, the earlier an intervention, the more likely it will involve crisis intervention and brief psychotherapy, and the less likely it is to depend, primarily or exclusively, on medication and expensive, sometimes frightening settings such as busy emergency rooms. Many people express a preference not to be on medications, whether it is based on stigma, fear, or the risk of side effects. While medications can be very effective in reducing symptoms and suffering, they don't provide skills and tools to promote functioning and resilience. And the long waits to receive any treatment can translate to drifting into repeated episodes and impairment, homelessness, crime, substance abuse, and even suicide. When we think of these things happening to a person like Shobha, who can't knock on traditional doors for help, the need for effective early intervention is clear.

More than a decade ago, Ashok did research on early case identification to reduce treatment delay in nontraditional, nonmedical sources of referral: churches, schools, etc. This led to a huge increase in people asking for help—not exclusively for first-episode psychosis but for a range of mental health problems and illnesses, from common problems like anxiety and depression to more rare illnesses like bipolar disorder and schizophrenia. He realized there was an ethical responsibility to apply the lessons learned from early intervention in first-episode psychosis more systemically to a broader range of mental illnesses. He also grew to believe that the entry to the mental health system, especially for young people, should be focused on problems rather than diagnoses.

For instance, Shobha's anxiety is real as she finds her way through some challenging circumstances at school and among her friends, but that does not necessarily mean she "qualifies" for a psychiatric label of an enduring mental illness such as generalized anxiety disorder. However, getting help shouldn't mean having to pass a diagnostic entrance exam! The barriers to entry to help need to be low, both to meet as many who are in need as well as to identify quickly those people who are struggling with early signs of a major mental illness. There should not be the assumption that every person with a mental health problem has a mental illness. That would lead to overdiagnosis and potentially a mismatch between treatment and need.

Indeed, Ashok is testing this out by looking at the combination of distress, functioning, and a clinician's general sense of the problem's severity versus more formal clinical diagnosis—one evaluation or the other may have a greater likelihood of triggering the correct intervention. Health care professionals and systems tend to organize around diagnoses, but is that the best way to deliver the right service at the right time? It is a legitimate scientific question that Ashok is trying to address. And from the perspective of patients like Shobha and families, here are the questions that count: Why do I feel so bad? Why can't I function like I used to? Do you think it's serious?

Ashok began to percolate the idea of AOM as a network beyond traditional hospital and clinic settings and truly integrated into the community when the Canadian Institutes of Health Research launched its Transformational Research in Adolescent Mental Health initiative. Teams from around the country prepared submissions for its unprecedented almost $25 million in funding, and an international panel adjudicated the applications. AOM was selected.

Before the funding was obtained, however, a huge amount of community building had to occur to construct components of a service system with input every step of the way from the young people and families who would be served by it. They asked for simple things—to be treated with respect, and to be treated not as a problem but as a person with a problem. This is a reflection of a broader theme in health care and its language—that we now talk of "a person with diabetes" as opposed to "a diabetic" so that diagnoses and illnesses do not define and sum up the person and that clinicians do not lose sight of the humanity of their patients. Despite the extraordinary reproducibility of symptoms of illness—which allows for the pattern recognition that underlies making a diagnosis—the unique impact of those symptoms on the individual is what leads to the "person with a problem."

In each community, a mapping exercise was done to chart all the resources that could be brought to bear to help young people. In most places, it is hard to aggregate this kind of information because there is usually no single front door to services. It takes leg work, detective work, and collaboration locally to discover all the existing clinics and programs and integrate the information for the benefit of clinicians (who sometimes are unaware of the full palette of services), patients, and families.

So what is AOM? It is a network of community-based centres in fourteen sites across six provinces and territories, from Nova Scotia west to Alberta and north to the Northwest Territories—a truly national initiative. Its essential components include: increasing the numbers of young people seen (with target numbers calculated based on science, using estimated rates of mental health problems and illnesses); offering to see young people within seventy-two hours of their asking for help; eliminating formal system transition from youth to adult when people turn eighteen (there is nothing magical that happens to people on their eighteenth birthday that changes their needs for consistent help); and engaging youth and families in the design and oversight of services. Finally, if a young person was assessed and determined to need specialist care by a psychiatrist, that would happen within thirty days. AOM is currently running in large urban centres, smaller towns, and indigenous communities.

What does an AOM site look like for a schoolteacher or guidance counsellor encouraging a young person to get some help? They can call AOM in their community and either send or, even better, accompany the young person to the site. Or a worker from AOM may come to where the young person is—that could be a coffee shop or even a car. And in the context of pandemic restrictions, services can be accessed online, by phone or by text. The sites themselves are completely apart from traditional hospitals and clinics; in Edmonton, it is actually located inside a downtown YMCA. The décor reflects input from youth to create a place where they feel comfortable. They are casual storefronts, and decidedly nonclinical. In the AOM site in Chatham, Ontario, there is artful graffiti on walls, relaxed meeting spaces that don't feel like clinics, sofas, and even hammocks rather than the usual office furniture. Youth, whether as concerned citizens or as service users or both, are engaged at every level in the organization, from governance to hiring panels for staff.

What happens when a young person like Shobha walks in without a scheduled appointment? She is seen very quickly by a clinician; waiting time is now being measured in minutes! If Shobha emails or calls, she will be offered a formal assessment within seventy-two hours. The initial assessment includes an understanding of the person's distress and an evaluation of suicide risk to figure out if it is an emergency, if referral to a specialist is needed, or if brief counselling is needed. Sometimes nothing is needed beyond reassurance; the goal is not to make every young person with problems and doubts a formal mental health patient. But so far, about two out of three people who actually come to AOM are seen as having moderate mental health problems that require further care.

If the clinician has decided the person doesn't need an ER or a specialist but still needs help, then that may be a single session or short-term psychotherapy. If other resources are needed, the community mapping helps to identify them. Indeed, creating these AOM sites has brought providers together who had not necessarily sat in the same room before.

In parallel and in the wake of AOM, there has been an explosion across Canada of very similar community-based programs under the general term of integrated youth services—and it is at the moment the single biggest transformation happening in mental health services in Canada. In British Columbia, the Foundry program already has multiple sites up and running, as do separate initiatives in Ontario and New Brunswick—reflecting the constitutional reality that health care is provincially funded and administered. Although AOM was established as a national research initiative across six provinces and territories, other similar integrated youth services are emerging with the support of both provincial governments and private philanthropy. The brand names differ—Foundry in British Columbia, Youth Wellness Hubs Ontario in that province—but the core components are the same. And governments are now enthusiastic about getting on board this fast-moving train. The various provincial initiatives are also developing a common language in terms of data and approaches, which should translate into an unprecedented ability to compare apples to apples across jurisdictional lines and to learn from one another.

Australia, which is rightly regarded as the birthplace of integrated youth services in 2006, now has approximately a hundred similar sites in their pioneering model called Headspace. Patrick McGorry, the Australian psychiatrist who inspired Ashok, is widely seen as the champion of this initiative. His country recognized his work in 2010, designating him "Australian of the Year" for his contributions to youth mental health. In 2006, its ambitious plan was to establish thirty Headspace sites across the country in two years. It has now more than tripled that objective.

Ashok would like to see every community in Canada have access to an equivalent of AOM well after the research study is over, with the creation of a national database that would allow Canadians to know (and to compare) how young people are doing when they get help. Indeed, Ashok and his team are helping communities beyond the AOM sites to set up similar operations. But it's not like a fast-food franchise; the model of care requires consultation with and adaptation to the local community needs and resources. It also requires a new and different workforce of clinicians beyond the traditional mental health professionals who can be easily trained up to provide the entry level of care, as well as trained peer support workers and trained family peer support workers.

The conversation about youth mental health has achieved a new prominence, whether from Prince William's and Prince Harry's support and action, the Bell Let's Talk campaign and philanthropy, Jack.org's national network of chapters and speakers (more on that shortly), and a general cultural shift toward candour about mental illness. For most of us as clinicians, a reasonable goal is to leave our patients better than when we first met them. For Ashok and his team, AOM is also a chance to leave a health system better than how they found it.

So how is AOM doing in achieving its goals? From the outset, AOM was designed to be evaluated in remote indigenous communities as well as in major urban centres, in recognition that there are many types of barriers to care and that responses must be tailored to the needs and cultures of the communities served. There is widespread recognition that the mental health needs of indigenous youth have not been well met and that tragic consequences like suicide are overrepresented. But there is reason for hope, and there are few better examples than the Eskasoni First Nation on Nova Scotia's Cape Breton Island. Hugging the shore of the Bras d'Or Lake, Eskasoni is the biggest Mi'kmaq community in North America. It has been an indigenous reserve for almost two hundred years, and its population of more than 4,000 people reflects in part federal government efforts to relocate and centralize indigenous peoples in the 1940s. Like many indigenous communities, the population is 50 percent young people, which translates into both opportunities and challenges. It means that half the community is passing through the age of maximum risk for the onset of a variety of psychiatric disorders as well as other mental health–related struggles.

I spoke with Daphne Hutt-MacLeod, a psychologist who runs the Eskasoni Mental Health Centre and who has been an integral part of AOM since its conception. Like many Cape Bretoners, including my aunts, uncles, and cousins from there, Daphne is fun and smart. She doesn't mince her words, and her enthusiasm for what she does is galvanizing.

Before AOM was even dreamed of, Eskasoni struggled with some tragedies and felt the need to transform. In 2009, there were eleven suicides among its young people, as well as seven infant deaths, and the community was engulfed in despair and loss. It attracted media attention and reinforced negative perceptions of life on a reserve. At the same time, government funds and the services that are supported by them were traditionally siloed into separate entities, leading to a lack of coordination and integration. People and community organizations got together to ask the difficult question, "How have we failed?" There were three separate mental health and social services for this small community, each operating independently. After months of review, it was decided to integrate services and leadership, and do so in a matter of days—"to rip the Band-Aid off," as Daphne put it. It was a shock to the system, but Daphne noted that after two months, both providers and people using the services realized they were better together than apart, all under one roof and one leader: Daphne.

She told me of a twenty-two-year-old man who presented to their crisis service in distress; he had a diagnosis of schizophrenia, was off his medications, was hearing voices in his head, but would not go to the hospital for his psychiatric condition. Daphne knew him and knew that he would accept help for his kidney transplant condition, though not for his schizophrenia. He agreed to go to the Cape Breton Regional Hospital for medical treatment; while there, the Eskasoni crisis worker facilitated his psychiatric care as well as his subsequent transfer to a rehabilitation program for his substance use. With the help he ultimately received, he ended up completing high school and community college. Prior to the service integration, he would have slipped through the cracks of more fragmented care.

So the momentum for change was already present in Eskasoni. And then Daphne saw the posting from the Canadian Institutes of Health Research announcing the funding for its TRAM initiative (Transformational Research in Adolescent Mental Health). She recalls letting out a scream of joy and thinking, "Oh, my God, somebody gets it; we have gotta be a part of this!" Daphne put the word out through the research network that Eskasoni wanted to be included and they were rapidly courted to participate in grant applications by national academic teams competing for the research funding, all of whom needed indigenous partners. In the end, Eskasoni was aligned with Ashok's network—one that emphasized those disenfranchised youth (indigenous, immigrant, homeless, involved with the law, etc.) who do not have easy access to the available mental health system.

AOM brought additional transformation to Eskasoni in the form of more clinical staff and an emphasis on research. Initially, Daphne balked at the latter, given the pressing clinical burdens, but then she found herself "eating crow . . . now I can't imagine having a service delivery without a research assistant." She knew she needed the evidence to show that system change works in order to sustain and expand the changes beyond the duration of a research project. Clinical systems were measured with rating scales that standardized information and quantified symptom severity. That helped to both crystallize problems and improve system reaction time in response to clinical needs. And having the data immediately available, rather than through the usually semiannual reports to government, pushed the system into more rapid response. If you have a thermometer, it helps to identify who has a fever and needs more treatment most urgently. It created red flags of disturbing trends that might otherwise have been missed, leading to faster clinical action. For example, when patterns of self-harm were identified among youth, Eskasoni immediately sought input from an expert for its frontline clinicians on the best ways to deal with the problem. As Daphne put it plainly, "Having information that allows you to turn on a dime? Now that's transformation!" She spoke of the importance of meaningful versus bureaucratic data, adding, "We want our funders to be happy—but we can't have any more dead kids."

There is a stereotype of some indigenous communities showing reluctance in embracing systemic change like this, but there was no resistance to ACCESS in Eskasoni. The community had both the experience of tragedy and the openness of leadership that contributed to a readiness for new models of help. The change included physical transformation, renovating an abandoned pool hall into a place where youth can access everything "from soup to nuts." In an effort to reduce stigma, it offers programming for all youth, not exclusively those living with mental illness and/or addiction. The programs range from pizza-making to archery to clinical care, family support, and employment counselling. Daphne describes it as the "fishnet model . . . get every kid you possibly can into the building"—and the youth who are either self-identified or identified by others as needing assessment and help are already there and the work begins right away.

Access to counselling is immediate, but access to formal psychiatric care by a child psychiatrist remains a problem. There is no child psychiatrist based on Cape Breton Island, which has a total population of 132,000. ACCESS cannot fix all human resource problems. Youth requiring inpatient psychiatric care have to be transferred to Halifax, a four-hour drive away from the support of family and community.

So far, the impact of ACCESS on Eskasoni has been palpable. From the beginning of the program, there were no suicides in the community—until two youth and one adult died by suicide at the end of 2018. But beyond those tragic outcome markers, there has been more positive change among youth, reflected by hundreds of youth engaging with new programs at ACCESS and getting the help they need.

When I asked Daphne whether she would have done things differently with implementing ACCESS if she had a do-over, she paused and then stated definitively, "Nope." However, she pointed out that the provincial government, which had provided a letter of support for the initiative, did not deliver as she had hoped. Regardless, other indigenous and nonindigenous communities in Atlantic Canada are coming to Eskasoni to learn how they did it, resulting in a spread of knowledge that is not centrally controlled by the government. AOM is a community-building initiative—both within and across communities—and works in ways that will endure after the research study is over.

Before AOM arrived in Eskasoni, data revealed to Daphne that the community was "first in everything you don't want to be first in . . . schizophrenia, suicide, diabetes . . . everything was through the roof from 2003 to 2009."

Implementation of ACCESS was "a breeze . . . no hiccups." The opportunities? Being part of a national project, meeting different people with different perspectives, and learning from them. At Eskasoni, they used a model that blended Western and indigenous ways of seeing the world; indeed, indigenous staff felt empowered with regard to their language and traditions within ACCESS more so than before the program was implemented. It also provided Eskasoni staff with the opportunity to interact with and learn from "highfalutin" individuals from other sites and jurisdictions—and see parallels to themselves. Ashok Malla was passionate about the inclusion of indigenous communities in AOM from the earliest conceptualization of the study. When Ashok spoke with the Eskasoni staff about problems in his native Kashmir and the impact of colonization, it made sense to them—"it has opened up the world to them." They are presenting their work nationally and internationally, whether at scientific meetings on youth mental health or gatherings of indigenous communities to address common problems.

For AOM across Canada, early data from March 2020 revealed that more than 6,500 youth had been assessed—people aged 12–25. According to the research of Ashok and his colleagues, as many as 80 percent of them were not having their needs met prior to AOM. Three-quarters of them endorsed moderately severe to severe levels of distress, and the clinicians who evaluated them rated two-thirds as having moderately severe to severe mental health problems. These are people who are struggling. More than 90 percent of these youth felt the service helped them with their problems and almost all would recommend the service to others.

By the fall of 2020, further data analysis revealed that young people who are at risk of marginalization—whether by racialization, sexual orientation, or poverty—connected with AOM in significant numbers. Most AOM sites met or exceeded the numbers of people they hoped to reach based on epidemiological projections of need in those communities. And for more than one-third of urban and rural non-indigenous youth, as well as for more than 70 percent of indigenous youth, AOM was their first experience of help-seeking, rather than an emergency room. Finally, over the four years of accumulated data, 83 percent of youth contacting AOM were offered an appointment within seventy-two hours. That is how access should be for a young person in distress.

The analysis of outcomes continues, but indicators like a decrease in psychological distress, an improvement in self-rated mental health, and an enhancement of social and occupational functioning all reveal significant shifts in the context of AOM engagement. Satisfaction among youth was high, and in perhaps the ultimate of endorsements, 96 percent of youth said they would recommend AOM to a friend. As for recommending AOM to governments, a preliminary economic evaluation revealed a dramatic return on investment—that every dollar invested in AOM services generated a return of $9.80 in terms of avoided traditional youth mental health service costs. The probability of AOM being a cost-saving intervention rang the bell at 100 percent.

Seeking help is one thing; being aware you might need some help is something else entirely. In 2011, a friend of mine called to ask me to meet with her friends, Eric Windeler and Sandra Hanington. Their son, Jack, had his life tragically cut short when he died by suicide in his first year of university. Eric had a career in logistics innovation in the automotive sector and also ran a start-up in e-commerce, and Sandra had been a senior executive in a bank. But when they had their fateful home visit from the police about Jack's death, their personal and professional lives were changed forever. I met with Eric and Sandra and their two other children about a week later as they reeled from the impact.

Born of this tragedy, a national movement has quickly developed. Today Eric is the founder and leader of the largest mental health movement in Canada targeted at young people and named in honour of his son: Jack.org. As early as Jack's funeral, Eric recalls feeling, "We've really got to do something." And he was committed to being open about Jack's suicide. Six weeks later, Eric started meeting with mental health experts, coupling his innate logistics approach with a problem whose contours he was only beginning to understand. He also began to discover the reality that suicide has affected many families but is often shrouded in secrecy, including the likely suicide of his paternal great-grandfather. "I always thought we were the happiest, healthiest family going," he said. Mental health had not been on his radar.

From there, Eric became a donor and full-time volunteer at Kids Help Phone for two years. Fifteen months after Jack's death, Eric had organized a pilot project involving thirty-six schools receiving 110 presentations about mental health to groups of students aged fifteen to twenty-four, to teachers, and to parents. However, the talks were given by Eric, then fifty years old, and two "young people" in their thirties. And because Eric insisted on evaluation, one of the biggest takeaways from the project was that the talks needed to be given by truly young people, the same age as their audience—who not only talked to but also listened to their audience. With this change, Eric found the turning point in his own grief, from depleted to energized. By 2013, Jack.org was legally established and its charitable status confirmed. I was eager and happy to serve on its board of directors from 2016 to 2019, riding its fast-moving train well after it had left the station.

Like the ACCESS Open Minds initiative, youth became intimately involved in the planning and development of Jack.org. When I visit its headquarters in downtown Toronto, I feel like a well-tolerated great-uncle by the young staff who are helping set up local chapters, train speakers, fund-raise, and conduct program evaluation. The organization is constantly modifying its approaches in the context of feedback from its youth participants.

Today, Jack.org has a presence in every province and territory of Canada, with well over two hundred chapters spread coast to coast to coast, usually in high schools, colleges, and universities but also in other places where young people congregate. This includes francophone, Inuit, and First Nations chapters. In high schools, there is usually a school staff person involved, but for youth over eighteen this is not the case.

What happens in a Jack.org chapter? A critical discovery was learning that one size does not fit all in terms of programming. The activities in a chapter need to reflect local context: resources, barriers, and needs. Chapter members are coached in how to explore these. Chapters range in size from sixteen to as many as 120 young people. Events are planned by the chapter to raise awareness about mental health in a way that fits their local communities, whether it is through starting conversations, fund-raising through fun activities, dismantling barriers to promote inclusion, or surveying the availability of appropriate mental health resources at their schools through the youth-led Campus Assessment Tool. Most of all, it's about the need to "make some noise" so that the silence around mental health ends and action ensues.

In addition, Jack talks remain an important component of Jack.org. As mentioned, speakers are young people, carefully trained in giving mental health awareness talks to their peers. In 2019, there were more than four hundred such talks across Canada reaching 60,000 students, almost double the preceding year's numbers.

Thirty Jack summits are held across the country each year to train and inspire young people to get the message out locally about mental health, encourage them to talk more openly, to join the chorus of demand for better mental health care, and to support and learn from each other. Overall, 250,000 young people will be reached via the combination of chapters, talks, and summits. The rate of growth has been steep—but Eric knows that there are roughly 3,500 high schools, colleges, and universities across Canada, and to date only about 10 percent of them have been touched by Jack.org in some way. Eric wants to triple that during his tenure—"We're just getting started." The organization is now known internationally for its work, including its commitment to open sourcing everything it has learned, so that other countries can replicate their work. To Eric's knowledge, no other organization outside Canada is as focused on youth engagement as a core principle in promoting mental health awareness. Jack.org is a true public health initiative, reaching out not only to those young people already struggling with mental health problems and illnesses but instead the "five in five" of young Canadians who are either at risk themselves or close to someone who is—literally everyone. It tries to teach them what they can do to help themselves, how to reach out for help, how to recognize distress in others, and how to help them.

Both AOM and Jack.org fill a huge need in youth mental health awareness, access, and care. Imagine if they, or other similar programs, working together, were the standard everywhere. At the beginning of this story, Shobha, suffering from debilitating anxiety and depression, felt isolated and afraid to seek help. There were few options available to her, all of which only increased her anxiety. Now imagine she had access to this kind of peer knowledge and support, learning that she is not alone and that others are committed to understanding her and helping her to get the help she needs. Imagine if Shobha then felt sufficiently encouraged and supported to be able to walk to the nearest community-based integrated youth service and, without an appointment or a waiting list, talk with someone right away in an environment that felt right to her, and then quickly get access to appropriate care. Why not?

Sometimes the standard response to unmet need is to provide more of existing services or to simply increase the number of traditional providers. Jack.org mobilizes youth in an unprecedented way as allies, supports, and advocates. AOM creates an entirely new and different context for meeting youth mental health needs. Both are committed to measuring the impact of what they do and having youth engaged at every level in their organization. It's a new way of thinking that challenges the status quo.

3

⟡⟡⟡⟡⟡

ELYSE AND BORDERLINE
PERSONALITY DISORDER

SHORT-TERM TREATMENT

◇◇◇◇

Extending a Digital Hand

"My moods change like a light switch, and over the littlest thing. My girlfriend says I'm bipolar, but she's a bitch." That's how Elyse responds to a general question from her family doctor about what is troubling her. At age twenty-four, she has been having difficulties in her relationships and within herself for almost a decade. At first, her parents downplayed the problem, saying, "She's rebelling." But what began as opposition and a snarky attitude has evolved into episodes of white-hot rage, and Elyse acknowledges that, among the many moods she experiences over the course of a day, it's that anger that is the most challenging for her. At times, it leads her to punch a hole in the wall or throw a plate, but just as often, it can lead her to cut her wrist or her thigh—not to kill herself but to distract herself from, or sometimes even punish herself for, the overwhelming feelings she experiences. She describes a feeling of calm rather than pain as she watches a thin trickle of blood arise slowly from a superficial cut. The calm can proceed to a sense of disconnection, where she feels outside herself.

What most commonly sets off Elyse, though, is the recurring challenge she experiences in her relationships. "I invest quickly and to the max," she notes, and it is rare that her partners, male and female (she identifies sexually as bi-curious), can keep up with her intensity. She always feels she has found "the one" and inevitably meets disappointment. Sometimes it is from an actual breakup, other times her partner is simply late or has forgotten to show up, triggering a deep-seated fear that she is alone and always will be. This leads to shouting matches and sometimes intense makeup sex. At the same time, though, she finds it hard to be monogamous. Impulses overtake her in a variety of ways, including casual sexual encounters, reckless spending, binge eating, and substance use. When she drinks, she is "all in," sometimes blacking out and finding herself in bad situations. She loves the rush of cocaine as a way of letting go at a party and having a good time.

And when the external noise subsides, she is left with a deep sense of uncertainty about who she is as a person and what her values and desires really are. In fact, she feels hollow inside. It's a sense of depletion and doubt, one that she makes desperate efforts to avoid because it is both painful and anxiety-provoking.

Elyse has had seven visits to the ER since she turned sixteen, usually after threatening to kill herself in the wake of a relationship breakup or conflict. Sometimes she has been intoxicated when she arrived. Each time, the feelings subsided and she was discharged from ER and sent home with recommendations to follow up with a crisis clinic. She has never consistently done this, easily frustrated by delays and feeling as though the clinic wasn't doing enough for her.

Once, when leaving the ER, Elyse glimpsed her hospital chart and saw the words "borderline personality disorder" inscribed multiple times. *On the borderline of what?* she wondered.

She found some answers through the one physician who is always available and always has a response: Dr. Google. As she read through the list of symptoms and the stories of others, for the first time she saw herself.

Her family doctor has tried to help her with antidepressants and anti-anxiety pills precisely because she spoke of how depressed and anxious she feels at times, but they don't seem to make much difference. She tried talking to a counsellor, but when he was late for her appointment, she stormed off and left him an angry voice mail, which she regretted almost as soon as she hung up.

Now what? she thought.

◇◇◇◇

Borderline personality disorder (BPD) rose to clinical prominence in the second half of the twentieth century. Its very name creates confusion about its meaning and often generates negative feelings toward the person given the diagnosis. It is one of ten personality disorders listed in the *Diagnostic and Statistical Manual of Mental Disorders, Fifth Edition*—the primary diagnostic tool for psychiatrists, known informally as *DSM-5*. Because BPD leaves people vulnerable to crises, it is likely the most common personality disorder seen in emergency rooms and family doctors' offices. It is characterized, like all personality disorders, not so much by discrete episodes of illness but rather by long-term ways of seeing oneself and interacting with the world that cause recurring problems in achieving happiness and fulfillment. People with BPD experience overwhelming emotions, a fear of abandonment, relationships that can be intense and conflict-ridden, impulsivity that takes many forms, a vulnerability to self-harm, and uncertainty in how they see themselves in terms of personal identity.

Like all disorders throughout medicine, BPD exists on a continuum of severity. It typically starts to show up in adolescence, often peaking in one's twenties and thirties, and then tends to subside, even without treatment, in one's forties or fifties. But just because the symptoms can disappear with time does not mean that we should avoid treating the condition—a lot of pain, stunted personal progress, and risk of injury and death can occur in the absence of intervention. And considering that BPD is a diagnosis found in 1–2 percent of the general population and in 10–15 percent of all emergency room patients, that's a lot of people who could use help.

BPD has a challenging reputation among clinicians and can inspire hopelessness, dislike, and avoidance. Even seasoned psychotherapists can be skittish about taking on such patients, feeling overwhelmed by their need, their instability, and their drama. But the evidence is unequivocal: People with BPD are helped by various types of psychotherapy (and much less so by medications). So how can Elyse get help?

To learn more, I returned to my first clinical supervisor in psychiatry during my training at McGill University in Montreal in 1982: Dr. Joel Paris. Joel is a leading scholar in the area of BPD, a previous chair of psychiatry at McGill, a former American whose idealism led him to serve in the Peace Corps, and a writer of some twenty books about important issues in psychiatry—especially BPD.

Many therapists are fearful of treating people with BPD and pessimistic about their outcome. By contrast, Joel takes a scientific, evidence-based approach. He is an advocate for the reality that people with BPD are treatable. His data shows us that they get better with (and even without) treatment, that they can get better without long-term and deep psychotherapy, and that we need to find the least intrusive, most efficient, and most effective form of treatment as a starting point. This challenges traditional beliefs, but Joel has always enjoyed being a science-based gadfly in defying professional dogma and tradition.

Joel was initially drawn to help people suffering from BPD by his experiences as both a physician and a therapist. He wanted to concentrate on the people whom he saw as particularly ill—and whom other mental health professionals feared—because of their chronic suicidal thinking and action. Prior to 1975, Joel didn't have a name for the diagnosis of these patients. But then he read a landmark paper by Boston psychiatrist John Gunderson, which showed that a consistent pattern of BPD symptoms could be recognized across different patients. That pattern formed the basis for diagnosing a disorder these patients shared and looking at both causes and treatments in a systematic way. Finding symptom commonalities among unique and different individuals is part of the detective work of psychiatric evaluation that allows for a shared language of diagnosis, even though the contexts of people vary widely. And making a diagnosis is a necessary step toward proving the value of a treatment.

Joel reinvented himself in middle age as a researcher after building a career as a clinician and teacher, and he became part of an international initiative to better understand people with personality disorders. He feels his best work to date was done after he turned sixty, which is inspiring for all of us. One of Joel's goals was pragmatic: He wanted to reduce the pressure on emergency rooms, where patients with BPD who are in a crisis often show up because of both urgency and lack of outpatient treatment resources. In all of the reading Joel did, it was clear that, in general, most of the benefit of psychotherapy comes from short-term treatment. So, over the past two decades, he has established clinics at McGill University for treating people with BPD using short-term therapy. Short-term treatment translates into more rapid access to help because of higher turnover rates, versus a model where a supply of therapists is rapidly saturated by long-term treatment. We know that in general hospitals people requiring medical inpatient care are often stockpiled in emergency rooms, receiving "hallway medicine" while awaiting the opening of occupied beds filled by people who don't always need to be there. The solution isn't more and bigger emergency rooms but rather more accessible and effective alternatives. Some patients with BPD are in the emergency room because there is nowhere else to go.

In 2001, Joel and his colleagues were among the first in Canada to offer a systematic short-term psychotherapy treatment for people with BPD. At that time, the dominant belief was that effective treatment was measured in years, not weeks or months. But "effective" treatment was hard to come by, whether due to filled practices or the antipathy toward people with this diagnosis. In a 2010 meeting of Canadian researchers and clinicians in BPD, Joel recalls that across the country there were year-long waiting lists and poor access to evidence-based treatments. There was an enthusiasm for developing newer approaches that led to some significant research funding and clinical trials; everyone recognized the status quo was not working. However, the wheels of science turn slowly, and going from proof of concept to change in practice is typically measured not across years but across decades. For Joel, it meant initially developing and refining a treatment approach that made sense to him as a clinician and appeared to help his patients, then subjecting it to more systematic research evaluation to see if his clinical impression was correct.

In the long journey between hatching an idea for treatment and having its worth confirmed through scientific peer review, Joel was able to demonstrate in a research publication in 2018 that twelve weeks of individual and group therapy for BPD was effective for the majority in a study of 479 people, with only about 10 percent of people coming back for more treatment. In the spirit of stepped care, Joel's system included both short-term treatment as well as an extended care clinic that provided care for up to two years for people with more chronic symptoms. And the waiting list for short-term treatment was at most a couple of months. Most people got better—a remarkable finding for a short-term intervention targeting a condition that had historically been perceived as both chronic and, to some degree, untreatable. Indeed, the editor of the journal where the results were published—a leading authority in the United Kingdom on personality disorders—felt that the British national guidelines on treatment for BPD would now need to be revised to include the benefits of short-term treatment. According to Joel, if the Canadian government would simply fund universal access to up to twenty sessions of psychotherapy per year for patients, there would be a net savings in health care, disability, and public assistance costs.

Learning how to accept, regulate, and tolerate emotions, how to put a lid on impulsivity, and how to deal with other people are some of the educational foci of Joel's approach. Joel describes it as "DBT lite," referring to one of the most studied forms of psychotherapy for BPD, called Dialectical Behaviour Therapy. DBT is the most evidence-based form of psychological treatment for BPD. Its components include mindfulness to help people be more accepting and able to tolerate being present, distress tolerance to avoid maladaptive responses to negative emotions, emotion regulation to manage the roller-coaster of feelings, and techniques for improving communication in and stability of relationships. It was rigorously evaluated in a large Canadian randomized controlled trial more than a decade ago. And as a clinician, I've witnessed its benefits in calming the storms that people with BPD can experience and providing them with safe harbour for overwhelming emotions and impulses. When delivered exclusively in a one-on-one format by a psychologist or other mental health professional, it can be expensive or lengthy, often lasting six to twelve months. While Joel's therapeutic approach acknowledges trauma in people's lives, it does not focus on it; instead there is a "get a life" component. The patients—especially the younger ones—are expected to be at work, or at school, or volunteering as part of their social rehabilitation.

Joel also acknowledges the benefit and power of the simple act of diagnosis, which helps put a frame on people's experience, legitimizing it. Having a term for their condition allows them to explore some of the resources in books and on the web, which can reduce the isolation and shame they often feel. In his experience—and mine—the majority of patients don't respond negatively to being given the diagnosis; that negative reaction is more common among clinicians! Reading about the diagnosis, identifying with it, and learning coping techniques can reduce shame and isolation while also making sense out of chaos.

Even if the research on these short-term interventions is so far limited, it still outstrips the evidence for the traditional (and wildly more expensive and less efficient) alternatives, such as long-term intensive psychotherapy and inpatient treatment. The prospects for people with BPD have improved greatly over a generation with regard to care and hope. Indeed, there is reason to be more therapeutically optimistic now than ever before.

Joel is not a fan of the use of hospitalization as part of treatment. "These patients need to be in the real world, in a social context—jobs, friends—and learning how to cope with it; otherwise, you're putting them in a bell jar," Joel told me. Decades ago, patients with BPD were sometimes hospitalized in Toronto for two years. Today, a stepped care approach—one that starts with the least intrusive, but still effective, intervention—is a much better way of helping people like Elyse get back to the lives they want to be living.

Montreal has the greatest number of programs in Canada for people with BPD. But everything that exists there can be replicated. In fact, the organization of primary care clinics in Quebec includes, in some instances, even less intensive group programs for people with BPD than the specialized services Joel has helped to create—exactly the sort of stepped care we need.

Of course, there will always be a subset of people who need more, not less, in the way of help, and everyone needs access to services that meet their needs. Throughout his long career, Joel has worried about the opportunity costs of treating patients: by continuing the long-term treatment of the patient sitting in front of him, who is being denied access to care? That is why he has tried to find the sweet spot of both providing enough care to get someone better and ending treatment with that person so another can be helped. It's about balancing individual health and population health as a single clinician.

But there's another option for access, and it does not include limited office hours, geographical barriers, out-of-pocket fees, or feeling like the initial assessment is an entrance exam to the highly selective school of help. And it is currently available in about 3.5 billion locations near you on earth: your smartphone. In what hardly qualifies as "breaking news," the number of smartphone users globally has increased by 40 percent in the last five years.

There are more than ten thousand apps related to mental health available for download, although, as of this writing, only twenty-two of them for depression and just nine of them for anxiety have been evaluated with our highest current clinical standard: the randomized controlled trial. It's a case of traditional science being unable to keep up with the pace of technology and entrepreneurialism. Ultimately, it may require a rethink of how we do scientific evaluation. While a medication once made is unaltered in its formulation for years or even decades, apps are in a state of constant update, making evaluations of earlier versions less relevant.

So far, the evidence tells us that smartphone apps for depression—an almost universal mood problem for people with BPD—are statistically better than doing nothing. And doing nothing is still an all-too-frequent outcome for people seeking help. The evidence is good but less impressive when apps are compared to traditional active treatments (if you can access them).

But there is one way that apps can perhaps improve things overall. In traditional, face-to-face care, people show up for scheduled appointments and are asked to recall how they have been feeling since the last appointment a week or a month earlier. Of course, their recollection is viewed through the prism of how they are feeling at that moment. When we feel depressed, anxious, or irritable, we selectively recall thoughts, feelings, and events that are consistent with that mood state. People with BPD, like all of us, can experience a variety of mood states across the course of hours, days, and weeks. Apps can randomly and irregularly ask you to rate and report on yourself between scheduled appointments, giving valuable information to whoever is treating you. It's no different than blood pressure or blood sugar readings that are done outside the artificial setting of a doctor's office. They reflect life in the moment, not life in the appointment.

There is a rapidly expanding field of monitoring through "wearables"—the Fitbit (or similar device) on your wrist and the smartphone in your pocket—that not only gather basic information about our steps taken or call history, but also track much more sophisticated data, such as where we go, how slow or fast we type, how we speak, and our virtual and physical destinations. And in the era of COVID-19, communities and nations are considering how this would help track the potential spread of the virus, with implications for the privacy we increasingly relinquish to technology. Amassing and making sense of all this data was inconceivable more than a decade ago, until the advent of something called "deep learning." Scientists use computational power and layers of data networks to detect increasingly complex phenomena. This is more than mimicking the way experts think. Machine learning has a limitless capacity for growth, to the point that deep learning can outperform human dermatologists in detecting skin cancers in lesions. So the next time you ask, "Does this mole look serious?" you may be texting an image taken with your smartphone to a virtual dermatology service.

Tom Insel, the psychiatrist who for many years led the National Institute of Mental Health in the United States, is a champion of digital technology as a means of improving how we monitor symptoms and deliver better intervention. Improving outcomes means better understanding what Tom describes as your "digital phenotype"—essentially, a profile of you via your smartphone, compiled both by passive monitoring as well as by actively measuring how you use your phone.

Tom and I have known each other casually for a number of years, running into each other at meetings as colleagues often do. So it was fitting that our several conversations for this book happened via FaceTime; we were able to not only hear each other, but make eye contact, too. It may seem like a small thing, but as social animals we communicate important information by seeing one another, something that technology now more easily enables.

Tom's own professional evolution has reflected his growing sense of urgency to translate knowledge into action. A well-trained neuroscientist who rose to the senior mental health research leadership position for the United States, he left that traditional path after many years of dedicated service to join Google's life sciences initiative, before moving to a tech start-up company called Mindstrong, which is focused on smartphones as a health tool. And in 2019, the governor of California appointed him "mental health czar" on a voluntary basis to modernize that state's mental health system—a state whose population exceeds that of Canada. He made a further professional pivot in leaving Mindstrong to cofound Nest Health, creating online peer support communities and therapists capable of providing single-session virtual counselling. This has been influenced by some Canadian work in Newfoundland, where a project called Stepped Care 2.0 demonstrated the value of such approaches in a research initiative led by Peter Cornish, formerly of Memorial University of Newfoundland; Cornish is moving from the northeast corner of North America to the southwest corner to join Tom's California initiative. So Tom's journey has taken him from the most fundamental levels of basic science inquiry, using complex and expensive technology, to detecting early signs of illness using a device that most of us carry in a pocket or purse.

Tom sees two ways these devices—which have evolved from pocket phones to pocket computers in a decade—can make a difference. First, they can both actively and passively measure such basic functions as sleep, physical movement, and even keystroke and scrolling patterns, which may allow for early detection of someone with a known psychiatric disorder getting ill again. Our functioning and activity can change in characteristic ways in psychiatric illness before the full symptoms emerge, an early warning system that can alert clinicians well before the next appointment—and even before the patient may be fully aware of the changes. Slower response times to texts and emails, decreased physical activity, more sleep disruption—all of these can be indicators of change in functioning and behaviour that need clinical follow-up. Monitoring yourself is like watching paint dry or grass grow; it's hard to pick up on changes until they are big. While some people are acutely sensitive to minor variations in how they feel and function, many of us are oblivious until there has been a major change for the worse. Knowing sooner can mean acting sooner. Second, apps will allow clinicians to integrate therapies with machine learning to personalize and contextualize help, which, in turn, allows for treatment without a human therapist. For instance, a change in sleep pattern detected by a smartphone may trigger the use of one of the existing apps that are successful at treating sleep difficulties. That app may then apply a proven combination of teaching proper sleep hygiene and providing cognitive behavioural therapy.

Unfortunately, in the high-stakes world of technology start-ups, Mindstrong had its own pivot since Tom and I first spoke about digital phenotyping, and the company has shifted from that type of passive assessment into more care delivery, reflecting marketplace demand in the private sector. But Tom still holds out hope that digital phenotyping, especially when it triggers active clinical intervention, will make a difference. In the mercurial world of Silicon Valley, it is impossible to predict whether what seemed promising in 2018 will take root. Meanwhile, in 2020, two major clinical trials are currently under way in the United Kingdom and several European countries examining the role of digital phenotyping to provide assessments on the daily reality of patients with depression and bipolar disorder between appointments. These are publicly funded science initiatives. If successful, this could prove to be a portable distant-early-warning system for these potentially debilitating disorders. It could trigger early intervention based on patient need rather than clinician schedule.

When Tom began his research career, he was thinking about basic science inquiries; now he focuses much more urgently on real-world outcomes, like meeting people's needs as quickly and effectively as possible to reduce suicide rates, hospitalization rates, relapse rates, and improving recovery rates. That shift in thinking has helped Tom feel more aligned with the priorities of patients and their families, a vital perspective for any health care provider. The world—and the field of mental health—still needs the most fundamental levels of medical research, from the molecular to the genetic and beyond, but there is now much more emphasis even in this research on addressing the "so what?" question with regard to how it will ultimately contribute to the well-being of people. It isn't an "either/or" choice in advancing knowledge; we need both the data that will make a difference a year from now and that which will change things a generation from now.

Most of us have made a relatively rapid evolution in incorporating smartphones into our lives, and feel suddenly at sea when we desperately pat our pockets looking for them. And researchers have placed much more emphasis on the effectiveness of new interventions outside the rarified air of traditional and pristine clinical trials. The thinking is, for people who are already diagnosed, the ease of using a smartphone will help reinforce better habits for patients and provide more robust data for clinicians. And starting with this population makes the most sense in terms of assessing the feasibility and effectiveness of digital phenotyping; people are more willing to use smoke detectors or burglar alarms after they've had a fire or been robbed once; no one wants to have a second encounter.

There is still room for improvement, of course. One of the challenges Tom sees with digital mental health treatments is that, while initial access to resources may be better than in normal care, actively sticking with the treatment remains lower compared to traditional face-to-face approaches. However, in terms of digital phenotyping, the ability that newer phones and devices have to passively monitor a patient all day solves this problem. As long as the patient's phone is charged and on them, it is gathering data about the person that is relevant to clinical status and care—from sleep and physical activity to social interaction, always looking for predictive patterns.

Another challenge with digital mental health is some resistance among the "analog" human providers. A decade ago, if a conference of hotel operators heard about Airbnb, they would have likely scoffed. Not now. And, as a doctor in his sixties, Tom adds that, "the next generation ain't buying what we're selling. They grew up with Amazon Prime and goods being available at their demand." People have learned to expect things and services to be provided almost instantly—and why shouldn't they, when it is possible? Simply giving health care providers more raw clinical information won't convince them to adopt a new solution; many of them already have an ambivalent relationship with the increasing amounts of time they have to dedicate to technology and increased data availability. Instead, the digital tools need to filter the data to save time: a traffic-light-style dashboard that provides go/no-go options for busy clinicians.

And, unlike drugs that are developed for illness, there is a continuous and iterative process between app developers and a world of users. Apps are being constantly updated with the input of—in this case—patients, families, and health care providers. This constant modification, which makes an app exquisitely responsive to feedback, makes it hard for scientists and regulatory bodies like Health Canada and the Food and Drug Administration in the United States to evaluate those moving targets. So not only do our treatment methods need to evolve but also our methods for evaluating treatment. It is currently a bit of a Wild West tech environment where the rules and regulations have not yet been entirely figured out the way they have been for prescription drugs. And little tweaks in technology can make big differences, unlike a pill whose chemistry and even shape and colour may be fixed for the duration of the patent on a drug that extends over many years.

Tom lamented that our thinking about apps in health care may be stuck in the "one bug, one drug" model of antibiotic development, where bringing a new drug to market could take a decade of development and testing, followed by another decade of patent protection without modification. "No part of that is relevant to the development of software in the health industry," he said. "We have to rethink the whole way this is done, with more evidence from the real world."

While there are many mental health apps, there is a minuscule amount of regulation that would help build public trust. In the future, cementing that trust might come more in the form of *Consumer Reports* and TripAdvisor than federal licensing authorities. When it comes to medical technology, we are in the first inning of a long game, and the most transformative changes could be peer-based, rather than expert-led. In health care, as in many other industries where technology is creating a new playing field, the online community will be a major driver of change.

We discussed the privacy challenges and public trust issues associated with monitoring people. Many have expressed concerns that virtual personal assistants in their homes, such as those through Google and Amazon, are constantly listening, waiting for their "wake word" to be ushered into service. Where does all the voice data go beyond building artificial intelligence regarding the user? However, passive behaviour monitoring through apps such as Tom describes does not collect data about what you type, but rather how you type. It's not evaluating patients based on the content of their messages, but rather on factors such as how fast they type, which machine learning can translate into signs of a relapse of depression. Nevertheless, apps are a business trying to thrive on the web. A 2019 study of thirty-six top-rated apps for depression and smoking cessation revealed that, while more than two-thirds of them had privacy policies, more than four-fifths of them shared data with Facebook and Google for marketing and advertising purposes, and only half of them who did so disclosed this to users.

Digital phenotyping can best be considered as a mental health smoke detector. Of course, smoke detectors are of use only if there are also fire extinguishers. That means linking the information obtained through digital phenotyping to the people providing care, combining online and offline interventions.

Recent careful research reviews of all the clinical trials done with such apps have convincingly demonstrated that they meaningfully reduce symptoms of depression and anxiety compared to control conditions.

In 2020, a survey of the most popular apps available for depression and anxiety revealed that among the top fifty, just three of them accounted for 90 percent of the downloads (10,000 in one month), daily active users, and monthly users. People are often skeptical of the idea that an app could relate to or "get" them. I encourage them to take one of the freely available apps, such as Woebot or Wysa, for a test drive. I did so for the first time in 2017, installing Wysa (one of the top three in popularity) on my phone and testing it by simulating the reactions of an angry, impulsive young man. In the app, I sent text messages to what I knew was an artificial intelligence bot and saw the blinking dots indicating the app was formulating a response, which appeared moments later. The app took some time to respond, and I wondered if an impatient, impulsive user might grow frustrated with the response time.

Later, I spoke with Jo Aggarwal, the co-inventor of Wysa, whom I had first met in person at a conference on digital psychiatry in England in 2017. Over a FaceTime call to her in Bangalore, India, two years later, I described my experience of waiting for the app's response to my messages. Jo laughed and said, "Yes, we had to reverse-engineer that. We introduced a delay so that the user would feel that Wysa is thinking about a response. In fact, with AI, the result is immediate." It was a little humiliating as a mental health professional to realize that the AI needed to be slowed down to come across as more human. And, of course, an app is never distracted from a patient by thinking about picking up dry cleaning later that day or wondering what that belly twinge could mean.

Everything that Wysa "says" is designed with and approved by clinical psychologists. It's built to pick up on nuances so that the machine decision-making can be more sophisticated. For example, grief is expressed very differently from depression, and each requires a very different therapeutic response; one size cannot fit all. Machines can learn the difference, as well as learn to recognize signs that someone may be in crisis or suicidal and connect them with help lines and self-harm prevention apps.

Wysa's avatar is a penguin, that monogamous bird who doesn't fly but is adept at both being on the ground and exploring the murkier area under the water's surface. In that sense, the penguin is a loyal partner who is adept at being both sure-footed on terra firma and ready to clarify the obscure—just like a good therapist. Jo told me that it was selected in fifteen minutes from random clip art, without much conscious forethought or design. It turned out that users loved it, including its genderless and body-positive status; Wysa has a significant LGBTQ following. Further, some people feel emotionally connected to the penguin and even do tribute videos to it.

When Wysa was developed, its target audience was the hundreds of millions of people in India in rural settings, far from mental health centres but near phones. But since its release, it has penetrated urban markets where barriers other than geography can prevent people from accessing help. Wysa has more than 1.9 million users and is growing at a rate of 20 percent per month. It is being used in more than sixty countries, but the predominance of use is in North America and the United Kingdom, reflecting its English language. However, Hindi and Spanish versions are coming to market.

Jo and her husband and cofounder, Ramakant Vempati, wanted Wysa to do more than simply dispense cognitive behavioural therapy (CBT); they wanted it to be "a good listener," an app that encourages people to feel comfortable disclosing difficult information. And in the pace of real-world app evolution and refinement, Jo notes that "each month we get better and better." The AI chat bot is free, but Wysa offers an additional paid option of text-based interaction with a coach, typically an experienced clinical psychologist in India who has had additional training in how to interact through text. There is ongoing monitoring as well, both to ensure clinical and efficiency standards and to protect personal information.

Two years after its 2016 release, Wysa had been used by 500,000 users, but it was still managed by a team of just five people in Bangalore, India—infinitely cheaper than the cost of such an operation in Silicon Valley. Two years later, the number of users more than doubled again. In addition to clinical psychologists who vet the quality and appropriateness of the content, former movie dialogue writers contribute to the expressive language the AI chat bot uses.

Jo taught me that an important measure in the app world is "net promoter score"—how many people recommend the app to others. In the first day or the first week, 70 percent of app users may drop off because they are simply checking out a free app rather than committing to it, much like people who don't get past the first chapter of a self-help book (or of Stephen Hawking's *A Brief History of Time*). At the same time, people may have obtained what they need from Wysa in the first four weeks. But 30 percent of people are still using it one month later. And in the United Kingdom, Wysa has become a preferred app for adolescents in the National Health Service, where it has been in extensive use.

There are two areas of growth for Wysa: language and voice recognition. This expansion of Wysa's capacity could make it the Waze of navigating one's mental state. This will allow people to talk with rather than text Wysa. And by broadening the language repertoire, Wysa could be more globally applied. But Wysa is far from alone in the world of mental health apps, and any book that tries to list them all is automatically out of date by the time it is published.

Another popular app is Woebot, whose clever name not only implies its mechanics and target but also triggers (for me, at least) images of cartoon character Elmer Fudd, who referred to his nemesis Bugs Bunny as "you wascally wabbit." Woebot is in use in more than 130 countries as a freely available mental health app that delivers a version of CBT. And it is the first in its class to be evaluated by a controlled research trial. Based on the data it collects, the app reduces symptoms of depression better than reading a book about depression does. It interacts with you, nudging you at times via text message, indicating it hasn't heard from you lately, and using humour appropriately—often a saving grace in difficult times. The language is plain, personal, and seemingly human. It is surprising to me that some patients tend to give Woebot and Wysa a gender identity after a couple of weeks, but it shows that the bot has become a responsive, remembering person to them.

I also spoke with Athena Robinson, chief clinical officer of Woebot and a Stanford psychologist, about the challenges of evaluating the benefits of a mental health app compared to a drug or a traditional psychotherapy. She noted that studies with Woebot take place in the hurly-burly of the real world, rather than the highly filtered and homogenized confines of a university clinic. They start with the assumption that all humans, like Elyse, have distorted thinking and trouble managing their moods from time to time and that all of us could benefit from learning some practical skills to help with that. With that in mind, Woebot can more accurately measure the varying levels of depression in the people it aims to help.

Despite the potential of apps, a download is not the same as an uptake. In other words, many people may use an app once, but consistent engagement is a challenge—some research indicates that three-quarters of users stop engaging with a health app after just ten uses. And when people do use them, it is for minutes, not a digital replica of an hour of face-to-face psychotherapy. Much like traditional mental health services, there needs to be better involvement of users in design and evaluation and better pairing with actual human services where available. As one of the world experts in this area, John Torous of Harvard, has noted, "Apps supported with human contact appear more successful than apps without."

That's why the researchers and software developers at Woebot have tried to create an app that is relational, one that is engaging and promotes a real alliance with the user that in turn promotes repetitive use. They have tried to develop a character for Woebot that Athena describes as "somewhere between Kermit the Frog and Mr. Spock," using humour when appropriate and cheering for the user when indicated. Amazingly, the app remembers what you have accomplished, whether a written record of thoughts that might otherwise go unacknowledged but have an impact, or the act of challenging one of your beliefs, or taking on an activity. Humans will disclose more to computer-controlled artificial intelligence than to a human-controlled computer. So the Woebot founders have tried to infuse the app with the kinds of human encouragement and curiosity that they use as clinicians to make users feel welcomed, heard, and not judged—critical elements of a therapeutic relationship.

With regard to privacy concerns, Woebot moved away from Facebook to its own applications to meet higher clinical standards for data encryption, and for research privacy purposes data is lumped together rather than examined individually.

Currently, Woebot sends out between one and two million messages per week to its users in 130 countries, even though it "speaks" only in English. It is hard to imagine a human workforce capable of that volume of interaction. Athena describes the mission of Woebot as nothing less than "radical accessibility to quality mental health care," including for people who are homeless or poor.

It is challenging for clinicians to stay abreast of the proliferation of mental health apps and know which ones to recommend. The American Psychiatric Association created App Advisor, an evaluation panel of experts to provide psychiatrists with important answers to questions about specific apps in terms of accessibility, cost, privacy, research evidence, etc. And a recent randomized clinical trial of an app for depression and anxiety confirmed its effectiveness.

Mental illness can cause people to feel isolated, regardless of whether they live in a sparsely populated rural area or a teeming urban core. In the face of that, these apps can provide an on-demand, 24/7 connection to an interactive, evidence-based resource. The Mental Health Commission of Canada has created a tool kit for all Canadians regarding e–mental health interventions, from telepsychiatry to smartphone apps. A demonstration project in Newfoundland and Labrador has provided preliminary evidence for the benefits of implementing an e–mental health strategy. There is a hunger in Canada for this kind of information and access; in 2017, more than 650,000 people visited the website www.ementalhealth.ca. In 2020, in the midst of the pandemic, the Canadian government launched its national portal Wellness Together Canada, focused on mental health and substance use, with a variety of self-assessment tools and resources. However, its listing of potential resources is not the same as implementing a stepped-care model that begins with the least intrusive, most available, and least expensive intervention—such as an app. The moment you open the app, you are not completely alone. And being alone is exactly what Elyse fears.

4

◇◇◇◇◇

RICHARD AND PANIC DISORDER

Self-Referral

◇◇◇◇

Good Things Come to Those Who Don't Wait

It came out of nowhere. Richard was twenty-three years old, driving his truck to work at a construction site, when he started to feel short of breath. He tried inhaling more shallowly and felt his heart pounding in his chest. He pulled over to the shoulder of the highway, gasping for air and wondering what was happening to him. A sense of dread overtook him—something terrible was about to unfold. The more his mind raced, the more he became drenched with sweat. He tasted vomit at the back of his throat, and as he sat panting in the cab of the truck, he felt light-headed, his fingertips going numb and tingling.

"This is it," he thought. He fumbled with his phone and called 911, his hands shaking as he punched the numbers. He whispered to the operator, "I think I'm having a heart attack." Paramedics arrived in a few minutes, moved him to a stretcher, and strapped an oxygen mask on his face. It felt surreal, as if Richard were watching everything unfold from outside himself. The paramedics seemed focused on their work as the ambulance sped to the hospital, while Richard's thoughts telescoped

ahead to the impact his death would have on his family, on the unfinished business of his life.

Hours later, after blood tests, an electrocardiogram, and a chest
x-ray, the ER physician broke the news: "It was just a panic attack. Here's
some Ativan to take if it comes back." But this wasn't "just" anything;
Richard had never experienced anything like this before and was still
fearful his life was over. He felt what he'd been through was being de-
valued by the physician. The message Richard got almost felt like disappointment—that the panic attack was "nothing" and the ER's resources
and time had been wasted. He felt embarrassed and unsure how to explain his absence to the guys he worked with, who frequently called each
other "wimps" and "wusses" when they balked or failed at aspects of the
job that required strength or endurance.

Over the course of the next four weeks, Richard had two more panic
attacks in the car, each causing him to exit the highway. He started taking alternate routes to the construction site that allowed him to avoid
the highway entirely. He was now often late for work, but the new routes
helped keep his panic at bay. The weeks turned into months, and Richard found that he was turning down opportunities for construction
projects where the only reasonable road to the job was via the highway.

He tried taking the Ativan, putting it under his tongue as the doctor
had advised. Within twenty minutes of taking it, he did feel calmer, but
it also made him woozy, and he didn't trust himself to drive his truck, let
alone operate a backhoe at the construction site.

Ashamed, Richard went to his family doctor. He was referred to a
psychiatrist but told that there might be a six- to nine-month waiting
list, and that was just for a one-shot assessment. "Doc, this is killing
me," Richard said. "I need something now." His physician gave him a
prescription for escitalopram, a popular antidepressant. Richard started
it, but two weeks later found that the immediate effect was a complete
blunting of his sexual interest. *I'd rather drive the side roads*, he thought,
and he flushed the remaining pills down the toilet.

◇◇◇◇

Richard needs help now, not six to nine months from now. Because his company has multiple construction sites across the city and its suburbs, he is often on the go and working in different places on different days. It is hard for him to get away from work during the day for medical appointments unless there is an obvious work-related physical injury—and his workplace is none too receptive to hearing about any psychological problems. He's a contract worker with no benefits, so paying the typical fees to see a psychologist in private practice feels beyond his reach.

In the traditional model of Canadian health care, we line up (if we can figure out where the line starts) for limited access to treatment: people sit on waiting lists for available, publicly funded services that are insufficient to meet demand. Those people who have either benefits provided by their employer or personal savings sometimes choose to seek expert nonmedical help, like that provided by psychologists and social workers, for which they have coverage or pay out of pocket. Doing so feels contrary to our national identity of universally accessible, government-funded health care. But for those with the means, it can be an attractive option. And who can blame them? For Richard, however, this isn't an option; even if he had benefits, they would typically cover only $500 per year of the costs of psychotherapy (the same amount often provided for massage) and this will pay for three to four sessions at most.

Richard has panic disorder—a well-recognized psychiatric diagnosis that includes recurring panic attacks that come on intermittently, suddenly, and unexpectedly, and that includes many physical symptoms such as shortness of breath, heart palpitations and chest heaviness, tremulousness, nausea, dizziness, and an intense fear. Panic disorder is one of the common types of anxiety disorders, a set of problems that include things like specific fears or phobias and the more constant and draining type of worry known as generalized anxiety disorder, which is often accompanied by muscle tension, restlessness, fatigue, and sleep disruption. These anxiety disorders as a group are the most common psychiatric disorders in Canada and globally, affecting almost 4 percent of the population but especially in Western countries.

Alfred Hitchcock's movies, heavily influenced by psychoanalysis, might have depicted such panic attacks as the adult consequence of a single traumatic event in childhood. Indeed, we are understandably drawn to the romantic idea that there must be an identifiable single explanation or cause when we are confronted with something that otherwise makes no sense. I wish it were that simple.

Anxiety, as a fundamental human emotion, can sometimes be justifiable and even helpful and appropriate. That is especially true in the context of the coronavirus pandemic. A national survey of almost two thousand Canadians at the peak of the first wave of infection revealed almost half of Canadians endorsed feeling anxious or worried, and only one in seven Canadians described themselves as feeling "normal." We are right to fear the virus, and that fear may lead us to make safer choices. Historically, from an evolutionary perspective, anxiety has galvanized people into action—or flight—when they are under attack. It can be a specific response to a specific threat. But when Richard has a panic attack, it makes no sense. Similarly, anxiety serves no purpose when it occurs in the context of the more continuous worry and vigilance that is generalized anxiety disorder: there is nothing specific happening to warrant such a strong reaction.

The traditional view of how to help people with anxiety is to tell them, "You have to talk to someone." In popular culture, that talking often looks a certain way—a warm, sympathetic therapist who listens more than they speak, sitting comfortably in an office that provides privacy and a safe environment for candor and confidentiality. Many people may assume that sessions will be weekly for an hour, and that it will takes months if not years of "digging" to get at "root causes" of the anxiety. And once the roots below the surface are exposed, the expectation is that the projecting tendrils of anxiety will wither, releasing the person from their ensnaring grip.

That works sometimes for some people, but for most people grappling with anxiety it is simply not an available, accessible, and affordable option. Richard cannot take the time to see a therapist once a week and he doesn't have the benefits to pay for it in the private sector. We need to look beyond our shores for alternatives that are solidly supported by evidence and anchored in a model of publicly funded health care.

A trip to England provides an answer. There, in an office in a converted house in Oxford, I first met in 2017 with Professor David Clark, the head of experimental psychology at the University of Oxford and the co-creator of England's biggest national experiment in better mental health services: Improving Access to Psychological Therapies (IAPT). A tall, friendly, but measured man with a shock of white hair, David is the embodiment of English calm. There was something straightforward and soothing in his manner as he explained what he and his colleague did—and why. It was nothing less than a revolution around how mental health care treats common problems like anxiety and depression.

IAPT began in England in 2005, when David and Richard Layard, an internationally renowned economist, wrote a paper that highlighted the national impact of mental illness on society and the economy. They proposed a treatment that would have no net cost if it worked—the costs of implementing the service would be offset by the savings to the economy from helping people get well and back in the workforce. They promised that outcome would be measured. The seeds were planted.

The British government took note—they saw there were real economic benefits to investing in mental health. But what made IAPT a success from the start was not only the buy-in from the government but also the initiative's direct appeal to the general public. They started with two pilot projects in 2006 and experimented with self-referral, as opposed to mandatory family physician referral, which had been the norm in England for accessing psychological services within the National

Health Service (NHS) since 1948. This was a revolutionary change. Within a year, the success of the program led the government to scale it up to the national level. It involved rapidly training a completely new class of psychological therapists—not traditional psychologists—and supplying them with standards, curricula, and supervisors. By 2013, the program had grown dramatically, assessing 600,000 people per year for treatment. That number has since gone up to more than one million people per year entering treatment, with targets to double that number by 2024.

At the core of IAPT is a rigorous emphasis on using brief and evidence-based treatment, what they call treatment "at the appropriate dose." And there is an insistence on measuring outcome at every single session—a simple rule that distinguishes IAPT from almost all other health care interventions. Grouped outcomes for every organization providing mental health care are reported publicly. It is also about matching people's needs to the intensity and type of treatment provided, rather than a one-size-fits-all approach to help. There are low-intensity treatments, like self-help and groups, as well as higher-intensity approaches, such as individual and couples counselling. Another significant systems game-changer is that people can contact IAPT directly for help, rather than having to be referred through their family physician as a gatekeeper.

Whom does IAPT help? The short answer is a long list: people with depression, generalized anxiety disorder, social anxiety disorder, panic disorder, obsessive-compulsive disorder, post-traumatic stress disorder, and health anxiety (hypochondriasis), among other conditions.

The IAPT Manual—which is publicly available online, another characteristic reflection of this initiative's transparency and accountability—outlines the details of the program. In providing a range of interventions from lower to higher intensity of treatment, the therapies mobilize an entirely new mental health workforce in addition to established ones. These are not psychiatrists, psychologists, or social workers, but rather psychological well-being practitioners (PWPs). The PWPs, who provide lower-intensity therapies, are often people who have an undergraduate degree in psychology but don't necessarily have previous experience as mental health professionals, so they are rigorously trained to provide specific, evidence-based treatments. The high-intensity therapists come from traditional mental health disciplines such as clinical psychology, social work, and nursing, and have to be able to provide multiple types of evidence-based treatments.

Based on the principle that you cannot change what you cannot measure, IAPT is keen on data collection—for accountability to patients, care providers, the government, and the general public. But it also values making choices available for patients, as well as reporting and reducing wait times for help. However, it's more than that; it's about having national standards and seeing if services stick to them. It may be surprising, but we don't have meaningful national standards in Canada for delivering psychotherapy. Imagine if in each province or territory there was one number to call to access evidence-based help, matched to needs and preferences, delivered in a timely way, and publicly funded and accountable.

IAPT has standards for how many people start treatment, for wait times, and for how many people actually get better. Let's start with how many people connect with IAPT for help. For 2015, the target was 15 percent of all the people in the community who had depressive and anxiety disorders, which amounted to roughly 900,000 people. Second, the national waiting time standards for IAPT state that 75 percent of people should have their first session of treatment within six weeks, and 95 percent within eighteen weeks. By 2018–19, 90 percent of people began treatment within six weeks. Finally, the British national recovery rate standard—or the number of people who finish their treatment with symptoms that are no longer severe enough to qualify for a diagnosis—sets the bar at a minimum of 50 percent of people treated. IAPT reached all of these thresholds.

In Canada today, that level of coverage would be a far-off dream. We don't currently measure wait times across Canada for accessing psychological treatments, but clinical experience suggests it is weeks to months to never, with little consistency. IAPT shows us that we don't have to simply accept the status quo—and that people like Richard can get help in a new way.

Because so-called universal access to services is not necessarily experienced equally across all groups, IAPT also collects and reports group data on who is being helped. They measure by diagnosis, age, gender, ethnicity, religion, sexual orientation, geography, and employment status, all of which helps to illuminate hidden barriers to care. It's a really important lesson for Canada, because the people who referred themselves to IAPT better reflected the reality of diverse communities than the people who were referred by their family physician.

Think about this for a moment. While we pride ourselves in Canada on multiculturalism and inclusion, we can't avoid the fact that, on the whole, different groups are treated differently in our society when it comes to access to care. The data are irrefutable. But a simple innovation, such as self-referral, can go a long way to address systemic inequalities.

Further, having services all over England means that IAPT can compare sites that perform well to those that perform less well, allowing the program to fine-tune and improve outcomes across the board. And here the lessons learned are not simply about patients but also about staff. Sites that provide personal feedback, supervision, and continuing education to staff—as well as providing staff well-being programs—have better results for the people they serve.

The data that IAPT collects also allows the program to identify those groups who are underrepresented among the people they serve: men; black and other ethnoracial minority groups; refugees and people seeking asylum; people with disabilities; people who are gay, lesbian, bisexual, or transgender; older people; and others. We would have a tough time in Canada figuring out in a systematic way who is not accessing such services, let alone devising relevant, targeted solutions. IAPT has done just that, developing guides for improving access and care for those underserved populations.

In IAPT, the best outcomes occur after an average of 9–10 sessions per person, with some people needing fewer sessions and some needing many more. It has measured and standardized outcome data on virtually every participant in treatment at every session—that alone sets it apart from almost all health care conducted at a national level. The results also fly in the face of cultural expectations of what being "in treatment" means for common mental illnesses such as anxiety and depression. Some people think that it can take many months or years to see meaningful results. By actually measuring and inspecting the evidence of our treatments, we might prevent systems of care from getting logjammed.

In Canada, the land of pilot projects, the government of Ontario has provided some initial funding for a more limited IAPT initiative, and Quebec is anticipating something similar. And in early 2020, the Ontario government committed additional funds to scale up the initiative within the province. But so far, there are no plans to roll out those projects into a national vision of what care should be for all Canadians coast to coast to coast.

Compared to Canada, England has more than a decade-long head start in this initiative, as well as a more centralized health care system that makes it easier to roll out standards and measure outcomes. But now, we have the opportunity to learn from the major successes and minor stumbles of IAPT; it appears to be one of the best-kept secrets from Canadian mental health care providers. When I speak to audiences of professionals around the country on the future of mental health care, only a small fraction of them has any familiarity with it. It's the reverse of a famous Canadian Red Rose tea advertisement on television forty years ago that showed British people sipping this beverage and saying, "Only in Canada, eh? Pity." We need to import this new British tradition and make it in our own unique blend.

That view is shared by Martin Antony, a professor of psychology at Ryerson University and distinguished researcher, teacher, and author. I first met Marty more than thirty years ago when we were both working at Toronto General Hospital, he as a research assistant and I as a newly minted psychiatrist. We got together recently to talk about innovations like IAPT and the need for more progress in access to psychotherapy in Canada. Naturally, neither of us has aged. But he has churned out books, largely based on cognitive behavioural therapy, which people with anxiety can use to help themselves, whether they have problems with shyness, social anxiety, perfectionism, panic attacks, or phobias.

Marty agrees with IAPT that self-help—whether on its own or accompanied by some guidance from a therapist—should be the first and simplest step in trying to help someone with an anxiety disorder. So why is that approach not more widespread?

One major barrier Marty points to is the overwhelming array of self-help options available, both in print and online. They have varying degrees of evidence to support them, so clinicians and patients don't know how to choose, and Canada lacks a national clearinghouse for recommended treatments. Simply reading a book or online article about mental health care is unlikely to get you better, in the same way reading about exercise won't make you fitter. Patients need access to professionals, people who will help them stay accountable for implementing what they've learned and monitor their progress.

Marty also notes that (despite his therapeutic optimism) change is hard—not simply for patients but also for clinicians and institutions. Twenty years ago, some therapists were unaware of evidence-based treatments for anxiety disorders, so there has been unquestionable progress. But he bemoans the continuing lack of measurement and accountability—the fact that, as a country, we have not committed to the important work of both gauging how people are doing, using simple but standardized instruments, and making that information available. It can be hard to teach an old dog new tricks—part of the reason that IAPT has developed a young and new cadre of PWPs.

Another obstacle in Canada is that we lack a national health care system like the NHS. Our federal government provides some funding to the provinces to support health care, and has in its most recent funding agreement directed specific funds for mental health services, but the services delivered are not nationally coordinated and standardized. We also do not have an evidence-based health care culture. Self-employed clinicians, as opposed to government health care employees, are tougher to compel to use outcome measures and evidence-based treatments.

So, what would Marty do if he was the mental health czar of Canada (like Tom Insel actually is in California), given that anxiety disorders are the most common psychiatric disorders and that access, standards, and outcomes are highly variable? He would start by allowing patients to measure their symptoms after appointments. The tool for doing this could be as simple as rating an Uber ride. He also wants to see a change in the culture among health care providers. Currently, therapists do a wide array of interventions with varying consistency and scientific foundation when what's needed is for them to adhere to standards and evidence-based treatment.

There is at least one Canadian example that incorporates values and approaches of IAPT as well as Marty's perspective. BEACON is a web-delivered version of cognitive behavioural therapy (CBT) in which patients receive a careful, front-end clinical assessment, followed by on-going messaging with a registered mental health professional throughout the course of treatment. It is available across Canada in both official languages through its website; its one-time fees are often covered by benefits plans, and in the context of COVID-19, the Ontario government made it freely available to its citizens.

BEACON is led by Dr. Peter Farvolden, a psychologist whom I have known for more than fifteen years, starting when he was a colleague at the Centre for Addiction and Mental Health (CAMH). He has had a long-standing interest in web-based assessment and treatment.

In 2013, Peter was approached by Sam Duboc, an innovative financial sector expert and cofounder of both Air Miles and Pathways to Education Canada. He wanted to help the development of a disruptive approach to providing therapy—not simply increasing the numbers of psychotherapists, but fundamentally changing the service delivery model to better address unmet needs, provide evidence-based treatment, and ensure excellent quality control. They looked around the world for models to import and found nothing that met their requirements, especially for people who needed rigorous, higher-intensity treatment with problem-specific approaches (rather than a one-size-fits-all model). And so BEACON was born.

In the BEACON model, patients begin by filling out an online assessment. When they click "Send," a calendar opens with available times to speak with a psychologist over the phone (which removes any geographical barrier). At the same time, the platform generates a draft report for the psychologist to review prior to the telephone interview. The psychologist can then use the phone call with the patient to establish a rapport and to probe further. When their conversation is over, the psychologist creates a final version of the report that's available to other clinicians as well as to the patient.

The next step is assigning the patient to an e-therapist, typically a young person who is more keen on and comfortable with a technological approach. The e-therapists are primarily registered social workers who get specific and ongoing training workshops in CBT. They work in an environment where they can consult easily with peers and senior colleagues about how to respond to clinical issues before they reply to a message from a patient—in the BEACON office, it's a large, shared space, like a fishbowl, where they sit together in front of individual computer monitors. It's entirely unlike the traditional setting of a lone clinician in an office who has to "say something" to their patient immediately. This allows for close and rapid consultation, case-based learning, and supervision. Like IAPT, there is a training curriculum for the e-therapists, and there is a commitment to getting them going quickly with patients.

Since its introduction in 2018, thousands of patients have been assessed and treated from coast to coast to coast in Canada. Its numbers have grown five-fold in its first two years and this is anticipated to double in 2020 with increased adoption by both public and private payers. And, according to Peter, 85 percent of patients presenting with panic disorder like Richard experience at least a 50 percent improvement in their symptoms, all through keyboard and internet interactions with a CBT program and a therapist. Of course, those results are not the reflection of a randomized controlled trial. But these evolving made-in-Canada clinical results are consistent with the rapidly expanding, international peer-reviewed research literature on this kind of therapeutic intervention, despite how different it seems from our traditional concepts of being "in therapy." No physician referral is required, patients can go straight to the website, and the cost is increasingly covered by employee extended benefits. It's not the same as a publicly funded treatment, however, so it will remain out of reach for a number of people. However, in the context of the pandemic, the government of Ontario announced a partnership with BEACON and another provider of online CBT to make help more broadly available to Ontarians in need. And it has been included as a form of treatment within the Ontario version of IAPT.

Where IAPT in England is accountable to taxpayers, BEACON has been privately funded, so to date the program has been accountable to those who pay for its services: individual patients as well as universities and insurance companies who cover treatment costs. "People have to know if the money spent is being spent well," Peter noted. While it may seem like an obvious statement, it is a profound one for the current reality of psychotherapy provision in Canada. BEACON has been set up from its inception to gather outcome data, therapeutic alliance data (essentially, the fit between the clinician and the patient), patient satisfaction data, therapist efficiency data, and other things that our public health care system is not currently able to do. A recent report of a thousand people who had used BEACON revealed the majority of users were aged 25–44 years, and anxiety and depression accounted for 85 percent of their mental health concerns. Two-thirds of users reported clinically significant improvement with treatment, about half reported a 50 percent or more drop in their symptom severity scales, and more than 90 percent reported satisfaction with treatment. Users are from over one hundred countries of origin and reflect the diversity of Canada. Those are more than acceptable numbers, even if the survey is not an arm's-length inquiry subject to the kind of peer review needed for scientific journals.

What would it look like for Richard seeking help for his panic disorder in a national system like BEACON? He would pay a single flat fee up front to register online. This is because he has no health care benefits at his job. In fact, if he had typical Canadian health care benefits from his employer, the majority of the entire cost of treatment would be covered. He'd then complete an initial assessment with a psychologist who would assure him he has a treatable problem and could explain how therapist-guided, internet-based CBT will work. Richard signs in and meets his e-therapist online the same day—a waiting list measured in hours, not months. He receives educational material and exercises on a weekly basis and can message back and forth with his e-therapist as much as he needs; the e-therapist usually responds the same day, up to a maximum delay of forty-eight hours. Richard can upload his symptoms and experiences immediately—a starkly different approach than "saving up" and recalling thoughts, feelings, and questions for an appointment every week or two. If Richard is able to put more time into the work, he can accelerate the course of his treatment. But if he's not making sufficient progress, his e-therapist can flag it, assess the risk, and trigger whatever intervention is necessary—all the way up to potentially calling 911.

For someone like Richard, with relatively recent-onset, classical, and uncomplicated panic disorder, a course of treatment with BEACON would be about six weeks. But patients have unlimited access to the platform and the e-therapist for twelve weeks, followed by forty weeks of unlimited access to the platform alone, with all of its tools, forms, homework, resources, and even the previous message interactions with the e-therapist. And no matter what, BEACON checks in with patients after three and six months to see how they are doing.

At BEACON headquarters, the biggest group of people was not the e-therapists, but rather the software developers, who were continuously tweaking and improving the programs. Their constant morphing of the program is very different than the more gradual accumulation of clinical expertise through the traditional routes. Traditional scientific and medical systems find it hard to meet "moving targets" in the same way.

With BEACON, the emphasis is on practical effectiveness. Peter makes the important point that while patient satisfaction is important, it isn't sufficient; there need to be good symptom outcomes as well. There can sometimes be a significant disconnect between high satisfaction, based on a patient's feedback about their experience, and actually getting better clinically. Peter and his team are committed to the latter.

Because BEACON is actively engaged with the private sector, it can draw on the expectations of private industry, which tend to be more demanding than the public sector when it comes to timeliness, efficiency, effectiveness, and accountability—not to mention better able to measure the financial return on investment. In terms of real-world effects, that can take the form of diminished sick leave and lower disability costs. That was the experience of Bell Canada, where an investment in the mental health of its employees was associated with a marked drop in short-term disability costs. Bell Canada not only focused its external philanthropy on mental health, through initiatives like Bell Let's Talk and the resulting investments in initiatives across the country, it also developed training for its managers and supervisors in better recognition of mental health problems and customized return-to-work strategies for employees who had been on sick leave due to mental illness.

While the private sector may be more nimble in these kinds of strategic initiatives, and more able to focus on and measure return on investment, there is no reason why the same could not happen in the public sector, much as is the case with IAPT, which is also expanding its digital services.

BEACON is not alone in the marketplace—there are other new programs emerging in Canada, although they don't use regulated health professionals and rigorous assessments in the same way. Currently, BEACON has e-therapists in every province and territory, as well as a bilingual platform and staff. This means registered and regulated mental health professionals in each of these jurisdictions are licensed to deliver diagnoses and provide e-therapy.

Eventually, BEACON could have an international reach, standing on the shoulders of programs like IAPT and harnessing the power of artificial intelligence to deliver high-intensity treatment with a small number of therapists. But in the shorter term, the goal must be to increase the menu of evidence-based programs available for treating specific disorders. Currently, BEACON has established protocols for depression, generalized anxiety disorder, panic disorder, social anxiety disorder, post-traumatic stress disorder, acute stress disorder, health anxiety, and insomnia. It will expand its services in 2020 to address obsessive-compulsive disorder, alcohol use disorder, and postoperative and chronic pain. Additionally, the pandemic has triggered the development of specific resources for frontline health care workers and first responders, including corrections officers. And BEACON, conscious of the diverse population across Canada, is actively trying to recruit people from different communities to be e-therapists so that they can provide sensitive cultural translation in their messaging. The possibilities seem endless.

There is so much unmet need, so many people who would benefit from mental health care, that BEACON has not been perceived as a threat by mental health professionals. The biggest negative reaction to BEACON has come from traditional therapists who view web-delivered CBT with messaging to and from an unseen therapist as a watering down of the complexity and richness of psychotherapy. It's worth noting that for the last fifty years this reaction has greeted new and effective psychotherapy advancements every time they've been introduced.

IAPT and BEACON represent examples of public sector and private sector initiatives to improve mental health care. We are understandably proud of the universal health care culture in Canada, the values it reflects. However, its realities currently exclude expert allied professionals from its basket of publicly funded outpatient services, and the system moves slowly in terms of innovation. Nature abhors a vacuum and so does the private sector. Even publicly funded health care institutions offer employees private benefits to cover otherwise uninsured services, including psychotherapy.

Both IAPT and BEACON ask the same bottom-line questions: Was it easy to get help? Did the patient get better? Those are the questions that should be guiding us all. As Peter notes, speaking as a PhD psychologist, "Show me where the evidence is that a PhD outperforms someone with a master's degree in social work in doing therapy. It isn't there." Results—clinical outcomes that are meaningful to patients—outweigh credentials.

And, of course, the old and new models aren't necessarily mutually exclusive. BEACON and similar tools have the potential to address less complex cases, thus preserving the advanced training of more traditional mental health professionals for the "tougher cases" in a stepped-care fashion. These new systems help bridge the current mismatch between clinical need and expert access. That means a better use of existing human resources rather than the traditional call to simply increase them—helping patients get better by working differently, rather than simply demanding more of the same.

Australia offers its citizens publicly funded CBT from psychologists;

England makes IAPT, with its range of mental health professionals, freely available. Canada lags behind. While individual provinces are making steps toward innovation, and while Canada has a national mental health strategy that calls for better access to psychotherapy, both in person and online, there is no coordinated national effort to move forward in any kind of lockstep. This is in part because of the constitutional reality that health care is a provincial jurisdiction. The Mental Health Commission of Canada, created in 2007, could play a vital coordinating role in moving things forward.

Innovations like IAPT, BEACON, and others can serve as a disruptive change to the system and even to the mental health professions. For Richard, it means the potential for two simple, but vital, things: not waiting and getting better.

5

◇◇◇◇◇

MARTHA AND DEPRESSION

PERSONALIZED CARE

◇◇◇◇

Genes That Fit and Magnetic Attraction

Martha is thirty-seven years old, a successful lawyer with two children under five years of age, living with her husband and live-in nanny in an upscale Toronto neighbourhood. She made partner in her Toronto firm at thirty-two and now enjoys a city-wide reputation as an aggressive litigator. Despite her successes, Martha has always known doubt and has experienced regular fluctuations in her mood, with a predictable tendency to feel down in October and November, as the days grow short.

This fall, in the absence of any particular change in her work or home environment, Martha felt more down than usual. She first noticed that she was waking up early in the morning, unable to go back to sleep after 5 a.m. It was at this early hour that she often felt her worst. She started to withdraw from social situations, giving a variety of excuses, and letting the phone go to voice mail. She admitted to her husband that she just didn't see the point anymore and didn't enjoy things; she felt like a sham and doubted whether she had ever really been happy. "I think this is the real me," she said. Without wanting to, she began to lose weight; initially, people complimented her on it and asked for her secret, but after several months, she started to look haggard and drawn. Her face took on a new flatness, seemingly unreactive to things good or bad. She even appeared to be moving more slowly. She became forgetful at work, had difficulty focusing, and was preoccupied with the idea that she had made a mistake, which meant checking and rechecking her work and consequently missing deadlines. Her colleagues tried to cheer her up with reassurance and suggested she simply needed a good holiday—"just go crash on a beach for a week; you can afford it." She began coming home early and spending time alone in her bedroom. One day, her husband found her organizing documents related to the house, investments, insurance, and the children into a file folder; she commented to him that they would be better off without her.

She considered speaking with her family doctor, but felt reluctant to drop her mask and reveal her distress. She made excuses to herself, fearing somehow that opening up would make it worse and would confirm her darkest fears. She also saw herself as an essentially healthy and capable person, who had bounced back after two pregnancies without any baby blues and had resumed her spot on the ladder at work. She had dutifully attended a lecture at her law firm on mental illness in the workplace, but thought of the content more in the context of her colleagues than herself—and knew that her being there reflected in part the need to accumulate annual continuing education credits.

Martha has a family doctor she likes and trusts, a supportive family, a network of caring friends, and financial means. Sometimes it is still not enough. Martha convinces herself she can ride it out, much as she has overcome other challenges in her life. She is a winner who has garnered recognition from her professional peers.

Nevertheless, she googles "depression treatment Toronto," and in under a second a list of twenty pages of clinics, individuals, and information websites appears on her computer screen that leave her at once overwhelmed and strangely uninformed. She feels she has no idea how to proceed in a way that protects her sense of privacy and her self-image. She knows intellectually that there are resources out there, including private ones she can easily afford, but she has no idea how to gauge their quality, trustworthiness, or appropriateness for her. She feels she is drowning within sight of shore.

◇◇◇◇

This is how it can start—for women and men, young and old, rich and poor. No one is invulnerable to depression, although across cultures and countries it occurs more commonly in women than in men; one in five women and one in ten men will suffer from depression in the course of their lives. It also tends to run in families. Most people don't have to look far to identify at least one relative who has been affected by depression. Typically, the earliest episodes are in adolescence and young adulthood, with a tendency to recur over the course of a lifetime—some people may have only one episode ever, while others experience them repeatedly. And sometimes depressive episodes may first appear when a person is a senior, which can lead to confusion between dementia and depression, especially as depression temporarily erodes cognitive functions such as concentration and memory (one of the key differences is that depression is highly treatable and thus a more optimistic diagnosis).

No matter how or when the depression manifests itself, treatment can make a difference. But people can be reticent about getting help for a number of reasons. Sometimes, people just don't know what they don't know. Even smart and accomplished individuals may not recognize that they're suffering from depression, especially when it clashes with their self-image of competence and coping. It's easier to assume there must be something physically wrong because of our sometimes-blind faith that finding physical causes leads to fixes. Other times, shame can hold people back. Many people may feel embarrassed to acknowledge that their minds and brains are not working properly. When someone as fortunate and accomplished as Martha gets depressed, she may think, *What right*

111

have I to feel this way? I've got it made compared to most people. I should be thanking my lucky stars.

If Martha were a lawyer in Australia rather than in Canada, things might be different for her. When the World Economic Forum issued its 2016 report on mental health, it gave examples across the globe of organizations that were getting it right. It included the prominent Australian law firm King & Wood Mallesons, which provides its staff with regular mental health awareness and management training sessions, designates well-being officers in its ranks, ensures its human resources staff is trained in Mental Health First Aid and accommodation strategies, and offers a psychological rehabilitation program. Opening the door to talking about mental illness and providing accessible help at that firm led to a surge in demand for help—but also a reduction in absenteeism.

And beyond this particular program, Australia is home to a "Resilience@Law" program that is a collaboration between eight major law firms and the College of Law to provide law students, lawyers, and judges with education about depression and anxiety, to reduce stigma, to provide self-care strategies, and to offer information about further support and resources. This program is a mandatory educational module at the college and it reaches 2,500 lawyers per year. Importantly, it includes videos of lawyers talking about their own experiences with mental illness and with what helps. Human stories—especially those involving people with whom we most identify—are more powerful than numbers and facts.

I have given numerous talks to groups of lawyers over the years about mental health in their workplaces. Recently one lawyer told me that he thought it was an important talk for his colleagues to hear but that it didn't really apply to him. Much as is the case in the midst of a pandemic, some people believe in their own mythic personal immunity.

In Canada, the Canadian Bar Association, the Mood Disorders Society of Canada, and Bell Canada's Bell Let's Talk initiative have developed an online course on mental health and wellness in the legal profession. It includes candid, courageous disclosure by the former presidents of the Canadian and Ontario Bar Associations of their own struggles with depression. However, as a frequent invited speaker at law firms and legal conferences across the country, I have found most lawyers to be completely unfamiliar with these made-in-Canada resources (when I ask for a show of hands), let alone with those internationally celebrated Australian resources. Indeed, when in 2013 the Mental Health Commission of Canada launched the world's first set of standards for occupational health and safety in the workplace (which have been heralded subsequently as the best in class globally), the Australian legal profession adopted them as their own. In Canada, not so much.

It is one thing to provide educational resources at a national level to raise awareness. But the old saying that "culture eats strategy for breakfast" applies here. Until and unless the local work culture changes, these excellent resources will not inform and, more important, help. It needs to change at Martha's firm so she can be encouraged and supported to seek help.

Even if a person does seek help, there are further, institutional obstacles. Limited resources can hold people back, and sometimes there's no clear path available. Instead of a robust mental health system, there is just a Google list of services and supports without design or logical sequence. Despite the range of services and experts available, many people resort to a default option, such as going to the family doctor (actually the best place to start these days), going to an emergency room (not an ideal entry point unless someone is in a crisis), or quietly asking a friend, "Do you know anybody good I could see who's taking on people?"

Finally, there is the stigma. There is a reality to the feared judgment of others. People may indeed look at you differently if they know you have a mental illness. While people talk more openly now about their chemotherapy for cancer and its terrible side effects, they are reticent to disclose psychiatric treatment. People fear the impact that disclosure might have on their work status or relationships. And they can also internalize the dominant social attitudes toward people with mental illness, so-called self-stigma.

Suppose Martha overcomes her self-stigma and goes to her family doctor—a woman she trusts, who delivered both her children and who is genuinely committed to her patients. As of now, there are no blood tests or brain imaging procedures that can reliably make a diagnosis of depression. It's a clinical diagnosis based on a pattern of signs and symptoms, and it can range in degree from mild to severe. So, the doctor may have Martha fill out some questionnaires and conduct an empathic clinical interview with her. The combination of Martha's scores on the questionnaire rating scales and the doctor's clinical impression would help both to gauge the severity of Martha's depression and, with repeat measurement over time, track changes in her condition—or even better, improvement.

Martha saying that her family would be better off without her and meticulously putting her affairs in order is a bad sign. In my experience, everyone who has been through a depression has thought about death in one way or another, from a passive "what if" in the context of feeling useless and a burden to others, to a preoccupation with methods that are highly lethal, like jumping, hanging, or guns. The clinician's job is to have that difficult and intimate conversation about suicide that the person may be very reluctant to have with anyone else.

Let's assume Martha's doctor has a good relationship with her so that they have that candid talk about suicide and Martha is open to getting some help. What would that help look like? Most people are treated as outpatients for depression, and the most common options are antidepressant medication and some form of counselling. Martha agrees to start medication, but decides to get her prescription filled at a pharmacy where she is less likely to run into people she knows. She's never been on an antidepressant before, so there are no good clinical signposts as to which of the more than twenty currently available antidepressants would be best for her. Her family doctor, then, prescribes the last one she had success with in treating another patient.

So the process of trial-and-error begins, which reflects a different kind of barrier to accessing care and recovery. More than half of people with depression will eventually experience some measure of improvement after starting antidepressants. But the chances that the first medication will completely relieve a person's depression are only one in three. Those numbers, when viewed by an individual whose depression usually includes an unhealthy dose of pessimism and helplessness, are often turned around: "The chances are two in three that this pill won't work." Treatment requires more than a pill; it requires hope, trust, and support. That's why medications are not simply couriered to people who complete a depression questionnaire and score in the "ill" category. Antidepressants are prescribed in the context of a therapeutic relationship.

Martha's doctor tells her that she doesn't know any psychiatrists who are currently taking on patients for regular psychotherapy, which would be covered by the provincial health plan. Indeed, she would be suspicious of a psychiatrist who had lots of availability—why is nobody seeing him or her? Instead, she gives Martha a list of psychotherapists, including social workers and psychologists, with whom the family doctor's patients have had good experiences. Martha doesn't balk at the fees, which range from $150–$300 per hour, because she has the means to afford it. But she wonders what the administrative assistants at her firm would do in the same situation. They get $500 per year in benefits for counselling, which would only cover several sessions.

Interestingly, the tide is starting to shift around psychotherapy benefits in the workplace as employers realize the enormous cost of disability due to mental illness. It is typically the leading cause of short-term and long-term disability in both the public and private sectors. As a result, such different employers as Starbucks and Manulife Insurance have raised their annual psychotherapy benefits to thousands of dollars per employee. However, for many companies their commitment to financially support the treatment of their employees for mental illness falls well short of what is needed—and is shortsighted in terms of the potential return on investment. The accounting firm Deloitte provided the numbers in a 2019 Canadian report that indicates clearly that investing in the mental health of employees makes money for the company.

But for Martha at least, antidepressants are the first step. The first medication Martha tries makes her severely nauseated and leaves her feeling both physically agitated and emotionally numbed. After two weeks, she stops it abruptly on her own and experiences "brain zaps"—akin to electrical shock sensations inside one's head—and a flu-like feeling for a couple of days as the medication works its way out of her system. These are well-recognized symptoms of acute antidepressant withdrawal when the medication is stopped suddenly rather than tapered, but they are new and frightening to Martha. Under the supervision of her doctor, the second one she tries helps her sleep dramatically, but it works too well—she sleeps eleven hours per night and feels sluggish during the day. After four weeks, she is about to start a trial of a third antidepressant, hoping for a Goldilocks experience of a pill that both helps her and that she can tolerate. It's a trying process for her and her doctor. "I feel like a guinea pig," Martha says, and on some level, she is right. Worse, deep down, each treatment failure reconfirms Martha's worst sense of who she is and what she deserves.

At the same time, Martha has started seeing a psychotherapist, a social worker with a warm and supportive manner who has a private office within her home and describes her approach as "eclectic and client-centred." It's not clear to Martha what that means, but she is relieved by the anonymity afforded by a residential neighbourhood compared to a medical waiting room in an office building. And her therapist provides a private and safe place for Martha to disclose her darkest thoughts and fears. The therapist quietly looks for themes and patterns that fit together to explain why Martha feels the way she does, all in hopes of providing a path forward. Martha finds it comforting to be with this empathic stranger, but the 167 hours between the weekly hour-long appointments leave her feeling strangely adrift.

Martha's husband, children, and family are perplexed by the changes. No one has told them what is going on. All they hear is Martha's admonition that they shouldn't worry. "I'm taking care of it," she tells them. Her professional colleagues are also in the dark, although the rumour mill at the law firm is that she's drinking or that her marriage is in trouble.

Martha wonders, as she treads water in the sea of her depression, if she is actually getting better or not. Monitoring herself is like watching paint dry and her perspective is distorted. Although she sees her therapist and her family doctor regularly, neither is measuring her symptoms in an ongoing way using any of the simple and proven rating scales to reflect severity of depression. Instead, both professionals are relying on their clinical experience, judgment, and memory. However, the term "measurement-based care" has taken on new relevance in psychiatry. Currently, fewer than 20 percent of mental health professionals routinely use such measures. By contrast, we expect the treatment of high blood pressure to be monitored and evaluated by the use of regular measurement via that tight cuff around our arms. Otherwise, how do we justify the cost and risks of treatment?

Researchers have identified multiple barriers to implementing measurement-based care, even though it may seem like an obvious thing to do. Patients may have concerns about where their data goes once documented beyond a conversation. Professionals may be skeptical that "the numbers" are more meaningful than their instincts or "global impressions," a technical term that fuses clinical experience and gut instinct to generate an overall sense of how a patient is faring. And health care organizations may not have the information infrastructure to make data collection both easy and useful.

However, researchers have also identified across multiple clinical trials that measurement-based care significantly outperforms "care as usual"—care without systematic tracking of symptoms using rating scales to both guide treatment decisions and gauge outcomes. This can be as low-tech as a nine-item questionnaire but provide the high value of a better clinical outcome for the patient.

Waiting to feel better can be especially hard for people suffering from depression. Martha is lucky: she has a caring doctor, a loving family, and the resources to afford the help she needs. Perhaps her luck even extends to physiology and she responds to the combination of the third antidepressant she tries as well as psychotherapy. But what if she can't get help, or the help provided doesn't work, or it's intolerable in terms of side effects and costs? What then?

It is sometimes said throughout medicine that when treatments don't work, "the patient failed a trial of X." But patients don't fail treatments; treatments fail patients. Imagine if, instead of sequential crapshoot trials of the many antidepressants currently available, there were biological markers to indicate which medications to try and which ones to avoid in terms of both side effects and benefits. It would save time, suffering, and cost. This is a different kind of measurement-based care than rating clinical progress on a standardized scale during treatment; it uses data from patients to guide clinicians toward picking effective and tolerable treatments for those specific patients.

This is the essence of personalized medicine. This is the twenty-first-century move away from one-size-fits-all in health care, and it ranges from understanding basic genetic markers to the simple effort of asking about people's preferences so that we can meaningfully incorporate them into treatment. What most people don't know is that we don't have to just imagine this. Some of the technology—and the move to involve patients in decisions about their care—is already here. Instead of our current off-the-rack options, what makes us unique as individuals—whether it's our DNA or our perspectives on illness and treatment—is built into a new partnership with physicians that allows for custom-tailored care. It is a shift away from the "I know best" attitude of health care providers to a more collaborative effort between doctor and patient.

Jim Kennedy is a psychiatrist and neuroscientist, the head of molecular science and head of the Tanenbaum Centre for Pharmacogenetics at the Centre for Addiction and Mental Health. When Jim and I first met in 1993, he was already balding—which means that almost thirty years later, he looks essentially the same, with perhaps some white mixed in to his blondish hair and aquiline moustache. He is one of the few psychiatrists I know who are comfortable in a lab coat because he spends a substantial amount of time with actual test tubes in an actual lab. He frequently looks bemused, almost impish, but he is bullish on innovation as a means of improving the lives of people with mental illness.

In 2004, while on sabbatical, Jim began to work on the role of genetics in antidepressant response. At the time, genetics was on the rise. Its role in breast cancer research had led to new, preventative surgeries—the era of using genes to manage risk and to personalize treatment was upon us. New antidepressants were being developed, but they often did not perform well in clinical trials because a proportion of people—up to a third of those treated—could not tolerate them. Jim thought it would be great if those people could be identified genetically in advance to see if they had the liver enzymes needed to metabolize the drugs. This kind of testing is called pharmacogenetics—understanding the role our genes play in shaping our response to medications. But the drug companies didn't want to identify people who probably shouldn't be taking their drugs, as that would reduce their market share up front. So they did not invest in Jim's research. Business trumped science.

In 2010, Jim finally found two important collaborators: a family doctor on the front lines of care who was willing to be part of a clinical trial, and an entrepreneur and notable philanthropist who saw the value of the research. The IMPACT (Individualized Medicine: Pharmacogenetics Assessment and Clinical Treatment) study was launched in 2011, screening for genes that affect the responses to drugs that treat depression, psychosis, bipolar disorder, and attention deficit/hyperactivity disorder (ADHD).

The simple goal is to increase the effectiveness of medication and reduce the risk of side effects. Jim's study doesn't just analyze people's DNA, though; participants also rate the severity of their symptoms and the side effects of treatment, as well as how well they perform at work. The result? The turnaround time from spitting into a tube to knowing which exact drug your body is likely to tolerate has been reduced to forty-eight hours, verging on Amazon Prime efficiency. And, of course, faster diagnosis and analysis means faster, effective, and tolerable treatment.

How important is this? Taking an antidepressant drug that's problematic for a person leads to more frequent health visits, more absenteeism, and higher drug and disability costs. A 2014 study compared people whose antidepressants were chosen through genetic screening versus treatment as usual. The "bottom line" results showed that, when choices were guided by genetic information, outpatient costs dropped and people stayed on the medication longer.

Imagine if your doctor received a report card on possible medications for you, clustered by colour based on your genetic profile—red showing the drugs your body isn't likely to tolerate, yellow representing the ones that might work, and green highlighting the medication that would likely work best, given your genetic makeup. What if that had been available for Martha? How drastically might her treatment journey have been improved? Systems like this could become part of the standard of care if the ongoing evaluations in Canada and other countries confirm their benefit. Antidepressants are among the most widely prescribed medications in Canada. With the tools we have, we could implement universal screening of people with depression to help choose the right drug for the right person at the right time.

A major American randomized controlled trial in 2019 examined the impact of pharmacogenetics on clinical outcomes in depression in more than one thousand people, using the same genetic test that Jim uses. All the participants had not responded to at least one antidepressant before entering the trial, and in fact the mean number of prior antidepressants tried unsuccessfully beforehand was three. For the subgroup of people whose medications on entering the trial were not congruent with their genetic profiles, when they switched to an antidepressant that was consistent with their genetic profiles, they were more likely to get better and less likely to be burdened with side effects. This is the largest study in the world to date on the potential benefit of pharmacogenetics. And a 2019 review of existing trials of this approach for people with depression indicated that those whose treatment was guided by pharmacogenetics had a 1.7 times greater chance of their symptoms going into remission compared to usual clinical care.

In Canada, a 2020 review of pharmacogenetics testing options revealed that while the tests are available in all provinces and territories, uptake is low and variability in cost (it is not publicly funded) and turnaround time for results (anywhere from two to forty business days) can place testing out of reach. And in the case of depression in particular, forty days to start effective treatment can simply be too late. Insurance companies are piloting the use of pharmacogenetics in mental health claims, because for them when it comes to prolonged searches for the right antidepressant, time is indeed money. At least one modeling study in 2020 (admittedly funded by the makers of the pharmacogenetic test) projected that by using the test to guide antidepressant treatment there was a potential overall cost savings of thousands of dollars per patient, from a Canadian public payer perspective.

This is less about new treatments than it is about using existing treatments better. Jim describes pharmacogenetics as "a game-changer, a revolution in the way doctors write prescriptions." It's one of the first major treatment payoffs of the decades-long neuroscience revolution. But the up-front cost for each test is still prohibitive, even though it may ultimately save money by more quickly helping people to take the right medication, feel better, and function better. The costs for each test will come down as they become more widely used, and the evidence base will continue to grow in its ability to improve treatment outcomes, but it's a work in progress.

Advancements in gene therapy will continue to improve our treatment of depression. But what happens if none of today's treatments for depression work for an individual? What do we do for the 30 percent of people who are being treated for depression but who are not responding to the treatments that currently exist? This isn't a small problem—that number of people with treatment-resistant depression adds up to 2.5 percent of the Canadian population each year. So as we improve our existing treatments, we also need to think about what other options have yet to be explored.

One increasingly popular alternative to pills and psychotherapy is magnets. This is not about people gradually pointing toward true north or being covered in iron filings. And it is not about magnet therapy, a pseudoscientific technique of placing magnets on parts of the body to supposedly improve blood flow or restore electromagnetic fields. The magnets we're talking about are a technology that ties into a buzzword in cutting-edge studies of the brain: neuroplasticity.

Jeff Daskalakis was the chief of CAMH's General Adult Psychiatry and Health Systems Division and codirector of the Temerty Centre for Therapeutic Brain Intervention until the summer of 2020, when he relocated to California to become the chair of psychiatry at the University of California, San Diego. When I was physician-in-chief of CAMH, Jeff was chief resident; twenty years later, I found myself reporting to him as my chief! Jeff is a product of Toronto's large and distinctive Greek community; I sometimes like to call him by his proper first name, Zafiris, which means sapphire. Jeff looks more hewn from granite than highly polished as a gem, though. He is relentlessly drawn to the new and bluntly passionate about improving our understanding and treatment of mental illnesses.

Jeff founded CAMH's Temerty Centre, where he and his team research new treatments for depression. One such technique they're providing and researching is rapid transcranial magnetic stimulation (rTMS).

The basics of rTMS date back to the mid-1980s, when a scientist named Anthony Barker and his colleagues in Sheffield, England, demonstrated the positive impacts of magnetic stimulation on the brain. The modern treatment involves passing an alternating electrical current through a coil to create a magnetic field. The coil is carefully positioned on a patient's scalp, and the magnetic field changes the normal electrical activity in the brain. That, in turn, affects the brain's nerve cells, causing them to release brain chemicals that are thought to be both part of the problem and part of the solution in depression, as well as chemicals that may inhibit erroneous, impulsive thoughts. Over time, these treatments can help the brain rewire itself, strengthening the healthy connections and reducing the damaging ones—neuroplasticity in action.

Until now, the ultimate form of brain stimulation has been electroconvulsive therapy (ECT), the oldest continuing biological treatment in psychiatry. It persists more than eighty years after its introduction for a simple reason: it works, and it works better than any other intervention, especially for treatment-resistant depression. Despite the benefits of ECT, though, it is an invasive treatment, requiring general anesthesia, triggering a modified seizure in a safe setting, and producing side effects such as memory disturbance.

There is a pressing need, then, for newer treatments that have fewer side effects and that do not require anesthesia, but that still lead to good outcomes. Lucky for us, rTMS does all of that. More important, rTMS offers legitimate hope to patients if drug treatments for their depression fail. And hope is one of the essential ingredients of medicine.

Jeff sees rTMS as "a leap forward." It's noninvasive, well tolerated by patients, and virtually free of side effects. Had Martha been able to have rTMS, she would have shown up daily at the clinic for about four weeks and sat in a chair for anywhere from five to thirty minutes while a technician positioned the coil over a carefully mapped region of her head and started the steady series of magnetic pulses. She would then walk out to her car, drive home, and get on with her day, not experiencing any significant side effects and gradually noticing a lifting of her mood.

Twenty years ago, there were just two rTMS centres in Canada; today the treatment is available on a limited basis in most provinces, but it remains largely unknown and inaccessible. And even in provinces where it is available, it is largely unfunded by the public health system. Why? Unfortunately, for the Marthas (and Martins) of this world who don't get better with trials of multiple antidepressants, the next generation of mental health professionals is not learning enough about how to use and value this relatively new approach. That's a failure of teaching. The people in power who make the policy and funding decisions have not made this technique more broadly available to Canadians. That's a failure of advocacy, despite a recent modeling study from Ontario showing greater cost-effectiveness and better clinical outcomes with rTMS versus ECT. There needs to be a national network of rTMS centres to help pool information and develop uniform standards. That's a failure of cooperation. As Cassius says to Brutus in Shakespeare's *Julius Caesar*, "The fault, dear Brutus, is not in our stars, but in ourselves." Finally, much as stigma has shrouded ECT for eighty years, it may well be that rTMS is not yet part of the necessary personal and public dialogue about depression, where it is more palatable to talk about psychotherapy and medication.

We need to be sure that the next generation of mental health professionals is up to speed on both new treatments and new approaches to choosing existing treatments. And we need to advocate loudly for the funding and availability of treatments that make a proven difference. Even with new approaches that have been shown to work, their clinical use has to be supported by research that teaches us how to make them even better for patients; there can be no standstill. Big knowledge requires big numbers, which means in Canada that there have to be links and information sharing between teaching hospitals within and between provincial boundaries; this helps to ensure that a person in Prince Edward Island gets the same standard of treatment as someone in Manitoba, while both contribute to a larger data pool to advance our understanding and treatment of depression.

In 2018, a major Canadian study appeared in *The Lancet*, one of the world's leading medical journals, demonstrating that a new, briefer form of rTMS produced comparable results to standard treatment in a fraction of the time for people like Martha. The next year, this same study was examined from an economic perspective; not only did briefer rTMS work as well as standard treatment, but it saved significant money and increased the time available for other people to get treatment. More Canadian evidence in 2020 examined the cost-utility of rTMS versus ECT in helping people with treatment-resistant depression. It found that rTMS was less expensive and produced better health outcomes as a first-line intervention in this population. And it is clearly less invasive and causes fewer side effects. The slope of the curve for validating and justifying rTMS is steep.

But, once again, from a stepped-care perspective, it is a stair that is all too often missing. Health Canada has approved rTMS for the treatment of depression since 2002, but fewer than half of Canada's provinces and territories have publicly funded access to this form of brain stimulation. We should be enthusiastic about a treatment like this, which does not require general anesthesia, does not trigger a seizure, and does not compromise memory while providing effective help for treatment-resistant depression.

Currently, we don't know for whom rTMS works best (a reality for many treatments in medicine). We do know, however, that our existing other treatments are sometimes not enough to relieve the pain associated with depression. We need more evidence-based options while we strive to see whether genetic profiles or symptom patterns will help refine our treatment selections.

There are groups in Canada hard at work on identifying other markers and tests that will allow improved individualized treatment. There has never been a better time than now, then, to move beyond saying, "This is what works for most people" to saying, "This is what should work for you." What helps other people—even many other people—is cold comfort if it doesn't help you.

Martha was fortunate that she ultimately responded to the treatments for her depression. But not everyone has such an easy path. Genetic testing will improve our ability to predict who will tolerate and benefit from a given treatment. And for the many thousands of Canadians who don't get better with the usual interventions, an expanded menu of treatments can ease the way forward. We have made-in-Canada proof that these approaches make a difference. It's time we used them.

6

◇◇◇◇◇

MANUEL AND SCHIZOPHRENIA

Training as Treatment

◇◇◇◇

Subtracting Negatives

Manuel is nineteen years old. He had always been a gregarious boy, active in sports and school theatre and typically surrounded by friends. Shortly after he turned eighteen, though, his parents noticed a gradual change in him. It happened over months, such that they couldn't pinpoint a moment or event when it all started. All they knew was that, one year after they celebrated his eighteenth birthday, Manuel was different—profoundly so.

He became more withdrawn, seeing his friends less often and spending more time alone in his room. He began to collect documents on religion and the occult downloaded from the internet and covered his walls in writings that were hard for his parents to follow. His sleeping pattern changed dramatically; he was up much of the night and slept through the day. He seemed increasingly apathetic, with no motivation to participate in the things he had so spontaneously enjoyed just a year earlier. His hygiene deteriorated, and he seemed both oblivious to the changes and resistant to pleading from his parents.

After several months, Manuel's parents began to hear him yelling in his room at night, seemingly in conversation with others, even though he was alone. He taped paper over his windows and insisted on eating only raw, unprepared foods. He became irritable and accusatory toward the people he had been closest to, frightening them and refusing their reassurances.

The final straw came when Manuel's parents found him punching holes in the wall, searching for "listening devices" and insisting that his parents knew what was going on. Their neighbour, a family physician, came to the house. He tried to speak with Manuel, who oscillated between anger and tears. Manuel then accused the doctor of being in on the conspiracy, too, and said that his only option was to kill himself before the "others" got to him. The doctor called the police and completed paperwork to allow them to apprehend Manuel for the purposes of an emergency psychiatric evaluation.

<><><>

Manuel's story mirrors that of many people who have been afflicted with schizophrenia or other similar psychotic illnesses. Schizophrenia affects about 1 in 100 people, men and women equally, and typically has its onset in late adolescence and early adulthood, although it usually hits a little later for females than for males. Schizophrenia is much rarer than common problems such as depression and anxiety, but it is usually more severe and persistent. The disease also has a greater capacity to derail a person's life and jeopardize the rewards of employment, relationships, housing, and even physical health and longevity.

The stereotypical image of someone with schizophrenia is a person huddled in a sleeping bag over a heating grate, disheveled and muttering to him or herself. And that may well be one of the faces of someone with schizophrenia, but there are many others, including people whose symptoms are under control and who are leading meaningful and productive lives. Such people are "invisible" to the casual observer, unlikely to trumpet their diagnosis because of the unrealistic fear it evokes in people.

While the exact cause of schizophrenia remains a mystery (like so many illnesses in modern medicine), it is hardly a "split personality." The illness is not well understood, despite the casual use of its name in everyday conversation: "The weather's a little schizophrenic today, starting with sunshine and ending with rain."

As with Manuel, schizophrenia can often begin with a gradual withdrawal over many months rather than an acute explosion of symptoms showing a divorce from reality, such as becoming severely paranoid or hallucinating. Because of that, it is hard to say exactly when such an illness actually "begins," and the lack of a defined starting point means that people suffering from the disease are diagnosed and treated far later than they should be. In fact, according to standard psychiatric guidelines, to diagnose a patient with schizophrenia, the patient needs to have experienced six months of symptoms. The reasoning behind the lengthy time requirement is that schizophrenia is not an easy diagnosis to undo. And some people will experience brief episodes of hallucinations and delusions without those symptoms evolving to a sustained period of illness. But that caution lacks sufficient compassion: six months is an eternity to the person suffering and their family.

Paranoia, especially when it reaches a delusional level, can exert a powerful grip. The disease can cement fixed, false beliefs in a person's head, despite evidence to the contrary. People suffering from such effects often take intervention to be a threat—they view efforts to help by well-meaning people through a distorted lens. Even the most random and benign aspects of someone's world—an innocent remark or gesture—can become loaded with ominous meaning and intent when schizophrenia strikes.

Hopeful parents may allow themselves to think that a person suffering from schizophrenia is "just going through a phase" and try to wait it out. Or they may be confused, uncertain of what to do or where to go for help. Worse, they might feel ashamed. While public awareness campaigns have made talking about depression and anxiety more acceptable, the same can't be said for schizophrenia. All too often, the hospital emergency room becomes the point of entry into care. Recent Canadian data shows that more than half of children and youth seeking mental health care via emergency rooms have had no prior contact with the mental health system. Surely there must be better ways for first contact that ease the burden on the system while also making it easier for those suffering to find care?

If Manuel is taken to the ER at a dedicated mental health facility, or even at most general hospitals, there would be an emergency psychiatric assessment to determine what is likely going on, if he needs (and is willing to accept) treatment, and whether he needs hospitalization or can be treated at home. Some such facilities exist and are able to provide both short-term care—with medications, psychotherapy, and family support—as well as more long-term assistance with school, work, and social reintegration.

But that specialized capacity isn't typical for most hospitals, clinics, and communities across Canada. Many Canadians don't live in the vicinity of such hospitals in major urban centres. There are some national organizations, such as the Canadian Consortium for Early Intervention in Psychosis, supporting advocacy, research, education, and clinical standards. There are also the Schizophrenia Societies that exists in each Canadian province, committed to providing support for young people nationwide who are facing psychosis for the first time as well as support for families and caregivers. And there are government-run websites, such as the ones for citizens of British Columbia and Ontario, that assist in making sense of what is happening and how to get help. Still, more is needed.

Specifically, we need better early intervention for psychosis. Psychosis is a generic clinical term that refers to symptoms such as delusions and hallucinations. The former are fixed false beliefs that take root and can be terrifying, such as the fear of people organizing to follow or hurt you. Hallucinations are sensory experiences without an actual sensory stimulus, such as hearing voices when alone that are talking to you or about you, often in a very negative way. While psychosis is an essential feature of schizophrenia, it can be seen less commonly in other psychiatric disorders, such as severe depression or mania, and also as a consequence of drug use, prescription medication, or other brain disorders. Regardless of the exact symptoms, early intervention means not simply the first response to a mental illness, but a range of services, including improved detection and diagnosis, better access to care, a multidisciplinary team, engagement with families, and a commitment to work with patients to evaluate their outcomes.

Early intervention for psychosis has grown substantially across Canada and around the world over the last twenty-five years. And yet, individuals and families confronting a first episode of psychosis are unlikely to know of such resources before they need them. At one level, it makes sense that people would be unaware of where to turn for highly specialized care for a relatively uncommon disorder—99 out of 100 people will never need access to this service. It's about the same frequency of occurrence as epilepsy for Canadians. But most people witnessing someone suffering a seizure would simply call 911, expecting an immediate and appropriate emergency response. Unlike epilepsy, with its sudden and dramatic first presentation, the changes in someone with psychosis can be gradual over many months before there is an acute eruption of disordered thinking and behaviour.

There are other barriers to knowledge as well, including stigma and the maze that is our current health care system. We know that early intervention is more effective than routine care, but such early intervention is not universally available in Canada, and we have no national standards for it.

How is it acceptable for a young person and family to be beyond the reach of these specialized and evidence-based resources at the onset of a

chronic illness, especially as the early stages are when we can most posi-
tively affect the course and outcome of a disease? Think how differently
we approach the diagnosis and treatment of diabetes in a young person
or the detection of potential cancers, before they derail a life.

It's one thing to be able to respond rapidly to an acute episode of a
psychotic illness, to extinguish the intense fire of hallucinations, delusions, and disorganized thought and behaviour. But what of the smoul-
dering embers, the charred remnants of the structure of someone's life
and functioning? Historically, this aspect of psychosis has received less
attention. It is heartbreaking to see someone's daily routine narrowed to
watching television numbly in an inpatient unit or in the living room
of a group home. The person with psychosis withdraws from the world
and, at the same time, the world pulls back from him or her—out of fear,
shame, or ignorance.

Medication is an essential and potentially transformative component of the treatment of people with schizophrenia, but pills or in-
jections alone are not comprehensive care. Medications are effective
in reducing or eliminating the "positive symptoms" of psychosis—by
which we mean additive symptoms such as the hallucinations and delusions the disease adds to one's life. But medications cannot replace what
the disease takes away. Patients and families are all too familiar with
those so-called negative symptoms of psychosis: the loss of motivation,
pleasure, interest, emotional reactivity, energy, or social engagement. In
many ways, social isolation and diminished self-care are the external
manifestations of these brain problems.

In recent years, we've also learned that the negative symptoms of
schizophrenia can be made worse by other brain-related challenges
brought on by psychosis. Psychoses can severely impact our brain functions, from the way we absorb, retain, and use information to carry out
complex tasks, to our ability to concentrate. Psychoses can even affect
memory. Diminished brain functions can lead to more obvious problems with basic aspects of self-care, such as poor hygiene and nutrition,

as well as challenges in maintaining relationships, succeeding at work or school, or even holding down a place to live.

Increasingly, then, when people speak of recovery from this illness, they refer not simply to the dampening of hallucinations and delusions, but rather toward reclaiming a meaningful and productive life and a valued place in society. So how do we best go about doing that? It's a question I put to Sean Kidd, CAMH's psychologist-in-chief and a scientist with a long-standing commitment to addressing the broad needs of people with severe and persistent mental illness.

Sean looks like a squeaky-clean folksinger from the early 1960s— slightly shaggy hair, a cropped beard, a sweater vest over a plaid shirt, and a gentle demeanour that radiates compassion and civility. He had started his undergraduate career in neuroscience while volunteering at a crisis centre and a homeless shelter; he subsequently completed his PhD in psychology, followed by postdoctoral training at Yale University, with a focus on youth homelessness. In 2009, he found his way to CAMH.

Sean has a particular interest in using cognitive remediation (CR) to improve real-world executive functioning, an umbrella term referring to the collection of brain processes needed to maintain relationships and function in society. Essentially, executive functioning is what allows us to handle complexity, solve problems, and be mentally flexible. Not surprisingly, the earlier that CR is delivered to people facing psychosis, the more likely the treatment is to have an impact. Indeed, various forms of cognitive remediation have helped improve real-world functioning in patients with schizophrenia for more than thirty years.

CR is often delivered through a combination of computer-based models and coaching, which are both labour- and technology-intensive. The core of CR is the online games that allow patients to repeatedly practice a cognitive task. The games target and train different aspects of how a person thinks—attention or memory or processing auditory information. The games help patients feel active, that there is something they can control, and that they are engaged. All of that helps to boost their self-esteem and hopefulness, as well as improve memory, attention, and problem solving. Even better, CR isn't necessarily hospital based, so the treatment can be provided in a number of different settings.

Of course, the games still need to be connected to the real world. "If you play a lot of Angry Birds, you'll get better at Angry Birds but not at dating," Sean says. That's where the coaching comes in. The coaching helps the patient transfer the skill from the computer game to a real-world task. So, for example, the computer game can be based on memorizing a restaurant order or recalling details of a voice mail message, and then a coach can help the patient perform that in a real-world setting.

So does every young Canadian experiencing psychosis for the first time get CR in addition to medication? No, which is a shame because CR is quite an effective treatment. When combined with job training and support in the workplace, CR can meaningfully improve patients' lives for years. Sean, like most experts in this field, believes that CR should be available for anyone with psychosis in Canada, the same way we would expect antipsychotic medication to be available for whoever needs it. Of course, not every medication works for every patient, and similarly, there will be some people who don't need CR or who don't benefit from it. But such outliers exist for almost all conditions and treatments throughout medicine, so that's not an argument to hold back the treatment. CR has the potential to be a part of a stepped-care approach to psychosis.

Before we can use CR to help people get the most out of work and school, though, we face a more basic task: we need to get people with schizophrenia to not isolate in their rooming houses. That's where cognitive adaptation training (CAT) comes in. If CR is designed to restore people with psychosis to a previous level of cognitive function, CAT is meant to find workarounds for enduring cognitive difficulties. For too many people with schizophrenia like Manuel, sitting in the living room of a boardinghouse or group home and staring at daytime television is a kind of mental prison. CAT can help them to break out.

CAT starts with a clinician assessing the type and severity of the cognitive challenges that a person is facing. The clinician then works with the person on strategies specifically targeting those difficulties. The training is one part basic organization (e.g., putting winter clothes away in the summer), one part offsetting cognitive challenges (e.g., using signs, alarms, and organizers to structure daily activities), and one part behavioural intervention (e.g., practicing casual conversation while ordering a coffee).

As an example, let's look at apathy, a common issue faced by people like Manuel. CAT interventions may emphasize prompts for a series of tasks, checklists to help the person organize what they have to do, and rewards for each job completed. If a patient is dealing with severe disorganization, CAT provides them with ways of reducing distractions and increasing order in their lives. Ultimately, the training is meant to help people reach more distant goals, like social engagement, by reducing barriers in their day-to-day lives.

What comes easily and spontaneously to many of us—everyday conversation—can be a significant barrier for some people with schizophrenia, even if they were previously good at it before the illness hit. Simple conversations can lead to the foundations of relationships that enhance our lives. It may be a casual chat with a server in a restaurant, a coworker, or a neighbour. A person suffering from psychosis may have problems decoding external reality from delusions, or may be distracted by hallucinations. Ultimately, he or she will likely experience disruptions of motivation that can interfere with what used to come naturally. Then the focus of CAT may be on social interaction rehearsal—this could be for something as seemingly simple as making a friend. Experienced clinicians have been gobsmacked by the gains made through CAT by some of their patients. Thanks to the training, actions that used to be incredibly difficult—making friends, dating, turning up for appointments, taking medication properly—became manageable.

The bad news is that the standard form of CAT involves nine months of intensive treatment, often with home visits, making it a sizeable investment in a time of limited resources. The good news is that Sean and his colleagues have come up with a much shorter version of CAT—one that takes only four months of CAT specialist intervention, with subsequent routine clinical care provided by existing case managers trained in the fundamentals of this technique. Sean has shown that, not only does it work, but that the benefits continued after the specialist intervention ended.

Sean is not a "techie," but he followed up his work in CAT with a foray into digital intervention. This move was inspired by a patient with schizophrenia who was using technology a great deal, making recordings with his phone to distinguish real external voices from hallucinations. Their conversations inspired Sean to look into apps, and he was surprised to find that, in contrast to the countless apps for depression and anxiety out there, nothing existed for psychosis. So, Sean worked with a health technology company to create an app that incorporates CAT, medication reminders, progress reports, text-based messaging for anxiety, helpful YouTube links, motivational techniques, sleep tracking, and peer-to-peer support. This technology, called App for Independence (A4i), also includes a feature that helps individuals with psychosis determine if the sound they are hearing is an auditory hallucination or is a real sound in the person's environment.

The features of this app are simple and useful for people trying to manage everyday life with a severe mental illness. But as noted in Chapter 3, there are many thousands of mental health apps; a download takes a few seconds but benefits require a greater investment of time. The challenge is how to make an app compelling enough for patients beyond its first or second use so that they continue using it regularly. In Sean's app, health care providers receive a progress report through a portal, and a dashboard update summarizes any activity since the last appointment. It's a wonderful idea with broad-reaching implications for meaningful feedback on progress in advance of the next appointment. Instead of asking patients to recall what has happened since they were last seen a month before, clinicians already have some data to work with, and perhaps even a new plan for further training.

But, again, reality intervenes. Many people with schizophrenia, even if they do have a phone, don't have a significant data plan. They may instead rely on free Wi-Fi in public spaces, which can limit how often they engage with the app. Part of what we need now, then, are the resources to connect people to this virtual help on a large scale—a small investment in phones and data plans with the big potential payoff of removing the invisible barriers to the outside world imposed by schizophrenia. That has the potential to improve the quality of life, functioning, and dignity of people with this illness.

As of mid-2020, the app that Sean and his colleagues within and beyond CAMH have developed now sits on my phone and I can see firsthand its straightforward user interface. Most mental health apps have been developed for stress, anxiety, and depression—admittedly a bigger market. But there is a small number of apps that, like A4i, are targeted at people with psychosis and have been evaluated in clinical trials. What they have in common with A4i is reminders around tasks, advice through text, and peer-to-peer support. However, A4i has novel features (such as the sound detectors mentioned above to help people distinguish external reality from auditory hallucinations). It works on a variety of phones and can be used with either a data plan or Wi-Fi. The app checks in with users twice per day, in addition to reminding them of appointments, social activities, and medication.

The app was carefully evaluated in a feasibility project published in 2019, funded by the CAMH Foundation. In the study, users of the app interacted with it on average four times per day. In our smartphone-obsessed world, this may seem like a small number of contacts. But for someone who is isolated, this has a different meaning. And the majority of users were satisfied with the technology in a one-month trial. This bodes well for A4i, and other apps like it that use prompts and reminders.

Once the constraints COVID-19 has imposed on clinical research subside, Sean and his colleagues will begin a major randomized controlled trial of A4i in people with psychosis, funded by the Canadian Institutes of Health Research. This may put CAT in the pocket of people like Manuel, whom the world of app developers, much like the rest of society, has largely ignored in terms of providing the tools, from technology to housing, to restore their functioning and connectedness.

It is easy to imagine that, five years from now, an app will be part of routine care for people with schizophrenia, especially if it helps to reduce rehospitalization rates. Already, roughly 90 percent of people with schizophrenia own cell phones. And the pace of development for new apps is much faster than it is for new forms of psychotherapy or drugs. At the same time, however, we have to go carefully so that we can ask the tough questions about whether such shiny, new tools make a significant, measurable difference. That's where scientists like Sean are so needed by everyone, tech entrepreneurs and patients alike.

Consider the possibility that most Fitbits and similar wearable tech are probably worn by people who don't strictly need them. For already health-conscious people, the step counts serve as gold stickers in their virtual notebooks. The idea that digital health tools and apps could instead be used to reach some of the most disabled and disadvantaged people in our society to improve their quality of life and functioning is exhilarating. It provides hope for clinicians and patients alike. Suddenly, proven treatments have the potential to move beyond the narrow confines of research centres and teaching hospitals into the homes—and pockets—of people struggling with schizophrenia day-to-day.

That excitement also fuels George Foussias, a young psychiatrist who is himself the progeny of two psychiatrist parents (possibly the only physician-parents not disappointed with their child's choice of a medical specialty). George has dedicated his career to understanding and treating the negative symptoms of psychosis as both a clinician and a researcher. He is modest but enthusiastic about the field of new technologies for an old disorder. And he runs the Virtual Reality and Behavioural Neuroscience Laboratory at CAMH while also serving as the chief of the Schizophrenia Division.

George initially became fascinated with psychosis when he saw the power of the brain to reach false conclusions despite all evidence to the contrary—the essence of delusions—and how people recover from that. But what intrigued him most, and what current treatments are worst at addressing, is the profound loss of motivation that can accompany psychotic states. What many of us take for granted—the drive to maintain hygiene, to interact with others, and to stick to schedules and routines—can be daunting when motivation is blunted. Low levels of motivation have been well documented in people with schizophrenia for more than a century. Too many times, psychosis leads down a dark path to nihilism in patients, and despair for families and clinicians. George refuses to accept that this "learned hopelessness" has to be a part of patients' lives.

George grew up when the first personal computers came into widespread use, as opposed to my fountain pen childhood. But now, as he stares down the barrel of his own early middle age, he sees young people with psychosis who engage with technology far more than he ever did.

George's first foray into the role of technology for people with psychosis was through virtual reality (VR), which he used to create simulated real-world environments for patients. His goal was to see how each patient acted and how well they functioned when they didn't have any biases and weren't consciously trying to minimize their symptoms to please a clinician. The best way to assess those things, of course, would be to follow patients around in their actual external environment. But George rightly figured that "most people would find that pretty creepy." Not to mention it would be overly time-consuming for clinicians.

So George created a vending machine shopping test in a virtual environment, one that looked very much like Ottawa. George's VR does not include the head-mounted, helmet-like experience that gamers sometimes use. Instead, patients sit in front of a panel of large monitors, which are less enveloping, more easily exported to other clinical environments, and, for some people, less nauseating.

The results from the VR tests, along with brain scans of the patients in them, helped George to understand some of the anatomical underpinnings of the motivation problems that people with psychosis face. There has been a long tradition in medicine of trying to localize central control of our functions and feelings in different regions of the brain—from the early 1600s, when philosopher René Descartes argued that a tiny brain structure, the pineal gland, was the seat of the soul, to pioneering work by Wilder Penfield at McGill University using neurosurgery to identify control centres. Apathy may ultimately correlate with dysfunction in a particular area of the brain or in brain circuits. And apathy holds us back from engagement and task completion. Using a VR task called the Multitasking in the City Test, a validated measure of people's ability to plan and carry out behavioural tasks, George and his colleagues showed differences between people with schizophrenia and health controls. People with schizophrenia had decreased virtual task performance scores, traveling further and with less efficiency. These findings correlated with problems in motivation and cognition. Using that knowledge, George created an eight-week training program for his patients to help them improve their mental stamina and ability to translate thoughts into decisions.

But do the skills transfer from virtual to actual reality? The answer is yes. Through this sort of mental training, people's motivation increases, their apathy decreases, and their functioning in various aspects of their external worlds improves. Patients start to reengage with work or school. Some critics feared that VR would worsen patients' tentative grip on reality, but the opposite proved true. VR provides a safe environment—one in which the risk of failure is low—for patients to "rehearse" new steps and strategies before taking them into the real world. In fact, the current VR assessment used by George's team takes only five minutes to gauge someone's motivation and related deficits—a spectacularly brief investment of time to begin to address a major obstacle in recovery. The potential benefits of VR to people with schizophrenia have been recognized in the recent peer-reviewed research literature, but its availability for patient care remains limited.

With the success of the VR treatment, George decided to go even further. Routine clinical practice for schizophrenia is still limited to asking people to recall how they felt about a certain motivation or activity, as opposed to measuring that patient's response in real time. So George and his colleagues built an app that does two things. It starts by acting as a scheduler for a range of activities in a calendar, linking them to real-world locations. Then the app tracks the patient's performance based on the schedule: Did the person go to that location? Did they arrive on time? How long did they stay? All of that information maps how social or isolated the patient is. It even provides a tool that prompts the patient to schedule physical activity and social interaction. All of the information is then fed into a web-based dashboard where clinicians can monitor the progress of the patient and identify where work needs to be done. All of this success in VR shows that, when built and delivered carefully and compassionately, new technology can help us scale up innovation in ways that will change patients' lives.

Today, when people present with psychosis, the focus is understandably on the hallucinations and delusions, with less attention paid to how the person's negative symptoms, such as problems with motivation, hold them back day-to-day. Hallucinations and delusions may be an admission ticket to treatment, but what limits people with schizophrenia in the long run is their impaired ability to be fully a part of the world, whether through school, work, self-care, or relationships. And those challenges are only made worse when coupled with inadequate housing, insufficient income support, and limited opportunity for community integration.

Imagine a future in which a patient's first assessment includes a video game on a tablet or virtual reality simulator. In fifteen minutes, the game or app creates a profile of the person that is instantly communicated to the clinician prior to their first face-to-face meeting. The physician can now personalize a treatment plan right at the outset. After the assessment, the patient uses an app to track his or her activity and receive behavioural prompts. Those digital tools could be a kick-starter in the patient's fight against hopelessness, activating and rewarding them to make small gains as a foundation for bigger steps.

It may be surprising that a chapter about someone with schizophrenia makes only passing mention of medications. It's not that medications are unimportant. Indeed, no one wants to go back to the 1950s and earlier when there were no effective medications for this illness (my father-in-law trained in that era of psychiatry and has told me terrible stories of both suffering and mistreatment). It's just that there have been no big drug breakthroughs recently (nor are there any on the immediate horizon), and no great evidence that the most recent generation of antipsychotic medications is superior to the previous one in terms of clinical outcomes. Newer medications may have different side effects profiles, but it is clear that the impact of these medications is minimal on the symptoms that preoccupy clinician researchers like Sean and George—hence the interest in CR, CAT, apps, and VR.

The uptake of such virtual reality and apps has been slow in Canada, although there is interest in the United States. Every day, Canadians use apps to pay for their parking, find the fastest route to their destination, review nearby restaurants, and monitor their own behaviour. But the integration of apps into the broader treatment of people with severe mental illness has been much slower, despite the fact that things move quickly in the digital world and that digital platforms are always being updated and improved (unlike us humans). Based on international evidence, the timeline for scaling up these interventions into standard clinical use is three to five years—an incredibly achievable time frame, but still, years away. George often says that, if he had a brother or sister with a psychotic illness, he would want them to access this technology now. As enthusiastic as he is about the value of antipsychotic medications, he rues the fact that, when it comes to cognitive impairment and negative symptoms, "we're still missing the boat." As Canadians, we need to do a better job of getting aboard.

7

◇◇◇◇◇

KIRK AND OPIOID USE DISORDER

Multidisciplinary Approach

◇◇◇◇

Get in the Fast Lane

It's one thing to ski for pleasure—the vistas, the fresh air, and the combination of exercise and gravity. But for Kirk, skiing was also about winning. He started in competition and training when he was eight years old and by age nineteen he was ranked nationally and participating in international races. He took chances and took tumbles, breaking a number of bones over the course of his racing career. He also had a couple of concussions.

But Kirk was determined; injuries would not hold him back unless he was in a plaster cast. So he soldiered on, using potent analgesics to mask the pain as he stood in the starting gates, poles planted, rocking back and forth on his skis until he lunged forward.

The pills were amazing. They had the capacity to numb the physical sensations of a body pushed beyond its limit, to the point that Kirk felt almost disconnected from himself, like he was floating on the fine powder under his skis. As his racing career grew, so did the list of sore muscles, broken bones, and post-concussion headaches he endured.

What began as episodic in his consumption of Percocet and OxyContin prescribed by his doctor gradually became more regular. And where one pill at a time used to work, three were now needed for the same effect. Soon Kirk found himself having to visit multiple doctors to get enough prescription pills to keep the wolves of pain at bay. Eventually, he wore out his welcome at physician offices, despite his stature as one of Canada's promising young skiers. This led Kirk to borrow pills from friends (it seemed like many had access to them) or buy them from strangers (also easily found, as many of his fellow athletes "knew a guy").

Getting pills began taking more of Kirk's time—and money. Friends started to distance themselves from him, telling him he seemed "out of it" at times. Meanwhile, the racing career that Kirk wanted, that the pills were supposed to help him pursue, seemed to be drifting away from him. His finish times lengthened, his rankings dropped, and his hopes of lucrative endorsements vanished. Making rent each month became a challenge as his money (like his mental energy) was directed toward one thing: the next dose. His racing career was effectively over and he had a new full-time job: addict. The pay was lousy and the benefits transient—just the buzz in the first hours after each pill. He was "fired" from his doctor's practice after forging a prescription and frightened as to what he was actually buying on the street after seeing a stranger in the final living moments of a fentanyl overdose. In desperation, he went to the nearest emergency room, knowing that the word "junkie" would immediately come to mind for the jaded clinical staff as they reviewed his chart.

◇◇◇◇

Canada and the United States are in the midst of an opioid crisis. It is about physical health, mental health, and death. The term "deaths of despair" describes mortality from suicide, drug overdose, and alcohol use and was invoked pre-COVID in terms of economic implications for the working class. The pandemic has made things worse. New models incorporate its effects on social isolation, unemployment, and economic hardship—and the likelihood for more deaths of despair. Based on three different rates of overall recovery from the impact of the pandemic, the anticipated additional deaths of despair ranged from 27,000 to over 150,000 in the United States. It is a staggering prediction. At the same time, there is hope everywhere that this crisis will trigger advances in treatment approaches for people with opioid use disorder by removing some barriers to help.

In Ontario in 2015, long before the pandemic, one out of every 135 deaths was opioid related, and among its young people it was a staggering one out of every six deaths. First responders across North America are now equipped with the drug naloxone to acutely reverse the life-threatening aspects of an opioid overdose. That can bring someone back immediately from an imminent death of despair, but the anguish itself remains unaddressed. Safe injection sites provide habitual users with a form of harm reduction, where clean needles, counselling, and even connection with a health professional are available. Physicians who glibly prescribed opioids (sometimes also called opiates) after being told by the manufacturers that the risk of addiction was low are now getting their education from different and less conflicted sources. And the manufacturers and marketers of these medications find themselves facing litigation, reparations demands, and bankruptcy. What can be done to prevent Kirk from becoming another sad statistic and human tragedy in the midst of this crisis?

Benedikt Fischer is currently the inaugural Hugh Green Foundation Chair in Addiction Research at the University of Auckland in New Zealand—his latest stop in a global journey that began in his native Stuttgart, Germany, followed by a PhD at the University of Toronto, and then a long stint at the Addiction Research Foundation before and after it merged with three other hospitals to create the Centre for Addiction and Mental Health. Although he is a researcher rather than a clinician, he is acutely sensitive to the tragedies that befall people like Kirk, and he has been an outspoken advocate in the scientific and public press for change for both better opioid control and improved interventions to help people with opioid use disorder.

Benedikt describes the current opioid crisis in Canada as being a bit like the 1994 hit movie *Speed*, where a bus has to maintain a high speed or it will explode. While nobody mistakes Benedikt for action star Keanu Reeves, he has some ideas about how to prevent the equivalent of a bus explosion for those passengers severely addicted to opioids. And there have been multiple feet on the gas pedal, including the overgenerous and even reckless prescribers of opioids in North America over the last two decades at levels higher than other countries globally. In Canada, between 2002 and 2012, there was a 140 percent increase in the amount of opioids dispensed. At its peak, almost 1 in 4 Canadians had an opioid prescription in the preceding year, and Canada's per capita opioid consumption was second only to the United States'. Benedikt led a cross-Canada study fifteen years ago to characterize the phenomenon of illicit opioid use. He thought there was an error in the data, until he realized there was a radical shift from illicit heroin injection to illicit oral opioids.

It has escalated steadily and is now almost a two-decades-old crisis, with the number of opioid-related deaths per year increasing annually and rivaling the number of suicide deaths per year in Canada at 4,000—a numbers contest that no one wants to win, and beyond the numbers, the tragedy of lives lost. Indeed, the death rate from opioids now exceeds those of car accidents and homicides combined.

Benedikt estimates there are several million Canadians now habituated to opioids, many of whom will have to turn to the streets for their supply. And they face double jeopardy: overprescribing got them into this jam, and current necessary constraints on prescribing may send them into withdrawal or abuse, even if those restrictions now prevent people from becoming addicted in the future. Further, the black market is responding to fill the void with illicit and increasingly often contaminated opioids that are completely unregulated and, as we have seen, sometimes laced with deadly fentanyl or other toxic and fatal by-products.

So what can be done? Benedikt supports the reduction and improved regulation of prescribing methadone and buprenorphine (opioids that are used to treat opioid use disorder by breaking the cycle of withdrawal and abuse), supervised injection sites, and emergency naloxone treatment. But he argues that these interventions won't help everyone in the long run. The missing piece in a comprehensive public health strategy is a form of safer opioid drug supply for people already engaged in high-risk use who cannot or will not sign up for other treatment options. This is a type of harm reduction that is equivalent to providing a clean needle rather than risking someone injecting with a used one—or providing clean drinking water to people exposed to contaminated water during an E. coli outbreak.

Supplying people who are seriously addicted to opioids but not open to the existing treatments (which are not always easy to access) with a safer opioid supply may seem like a radical idea—the long arm of the government feeding an addiction. Rather, it is considered as an emergency public health measure to prevent people from dying, but the stigma surrounding addiction feeds the neglect of this population. Indeed, the approach has been in place in Ottawa and Vancouver for several years, using the potent opioid hydromorphone, known by its trade name Dilaudid, with staff dispensing and overseeing the ingestion or injection of it. Dr. Jeff Turnbull in Ottawa, former chief of staff of the Ottawa Hospital and past president of the Canadian Medical Association, has been an outspoken advocate for a safer opioid supply for the homeless and people struggling with addiction whom he sees in his clinical work. It is a small-scale but important initiative. In August 2020, the federal government announced new funding to make a safe opioid supply available in Toronto for people with severe addiction to help them avoid dangerous street drugs. At the same time, the Public Prosecution Service of Canada revised its approach to drug offences, markedly diminishing the likelihood that people would be prosecuted criminally for simple possession of opioids. It isn't decriminalization, but you can see it from there.

However, Benedikt wonders about how to address the 1–2 million people across Canada estimated to be opioid dependent. He likens it to a vaccination program that only reaches a minority of the vulnerable population instead of protecting as many people as possible.

Benedikt thinks this strategy needs to be endorsed and led top-down, such as from the Public Health Agency of Canada and its provincial/territorial counterparts. This would be a big change not only in policy but also in culture and attitudes. Stigma persists despite political correctness, and the "morality dynamic" of addiction lingers, much as it did in the early days of HIV, especially when some considered its transmission the result of "immoral" sexual behaviour. Which politician wants to announce, "As a public health measure, we will provide people who are habituated to opioids with free opioids to protect their lives"?

There is a paucity of international examples of such exceptional behaviour to follow because no other countries have experienced the catastrophic opioid crisis that has affected North America. However, countries such as Portugal have decriminalized possession and consumption of illicit substances for two decades, driven by the desire to reduce HIV infection from injection drug use, with resulting reductions in incarceration, improvements in public health, and no significant increase in substance use. At the same time, Portugal introduced a broader range of treatment options for substance use as well as improved income support.

But we need not look across the ocean to see examples of such preventative policies. In other areas of public health, like injury prevention and infection control, the system provides proactive intervention to separate the human at risk from the potential harm. Just think of seat belts or flu shots. The failure to address the illegal use of opioids and its consequences in Canada may have cost thousands of lives—including potentially Kirk's.

And what would happen to those people who would be maintained on a government-funded, uncontaminated, and regulated source of safer opioids? If they are on public assistance, they would be less compelled to divert that money from housing and food into drugs. They would be less compelled to either commit crime or interact with criminals to sustain their dependence. They would be in more regular contact with health professionals committed to trying to engage them in treatment over the longer term. And they would be less likely to die in a back alley because of the use of contaminated drugs.

The majority of opioid-related deaths are among young people aged twenty to thirty-nine. People like Kirk. This has to change, with action that is both incremental and bold. And on this front, we have been failing for many years. A report from Vancouver's Community Chest and Council in 1952 on heroin addiction suggested that the federal government dispense heroin to people who were addicted to it, allowing them to lead safer, less precarious lives free of crime, and engaging them in rehabilitation. This was echoed in a 1994 review by a coroner in Vancouver. And then the limits to existing approaches were encapsulated in a 2020 publication on Vancouver's crisis, titled "Been there, done that." Almost seventy years after that first report, we face an opioid crisis that continues to escalate.

Mel Kahan is a veteran in the drug wars and has the gray hair and rumpled appearance to prove it. Trained as a family physician, he began working in addictions a half day per week in the early 1980s at the Addiction Research Foundation in Toronto. As his interest grew, so did his role there over the next nineteen years, including when he and I first met on the creation of CAMH in 1998. Like me, he recalls the "ping-pong" game of patients with alcohol use disorders and depression bouncing back and forth between the adjacent emergency rooms of the

Addiction Research Foundation and the Clarke Institute of Psychiatry. While Canada has moved significantly away from the separate silos of substance use and mental health care, their full integration at a national level is still significantly in the future. Mel moved next to St. Joseph's Health Centre, a busy community general hospital in the west end of Toronto. It was there, twenty years ago, that he established Toronto's first Rapid Access Addiction Medicine (RAAM) clinic—a concept that has since spread as an important component of a broader response to substance use disorders.

RAAM was a response to a broken system for addiction treatment, with the reality that people with substance use disorders presented to ERs in high numbers but there were no services immediately available to them. There were "psychosocial" programs, where the emphasis was on peer support and counselling with little role for medications; and there were methadone clinics with high volumes of patients daily and little role for counselling. So even within the field of substance use disorders, care was siloed. There were also significant divisions among those clinicians and organizations that opted for complete abstinence and those that allowed for harm reduction as well. But for all programs there were significant barriers to access, from waiting lists to complex assessments to a need for a certain level of stability and adherence to rules that were elusive for people in crisis.

The clinic was designed to be, like its title suggests, an urgent response that stabilized people, got them started on treatment, and integrated them back into family medicine care—"where they belong," Mel added. Mel welcomed these patients rather than avoiding them. That first clinic in the late 1990s was, to Mel's knowledge, unique and new. It accepted patients from ERs, inpatient units, and the community—and saw them within a couple of days to initiate treatment. The options that can be offered to patients in terms of medications to prevent cravings for and use of illicit drugs and alcohol have expanded significantly over the last two decades. But now, much as back then, the biggest challenge is patient engagement when patients fear being judged and endorse self-blame and hopelessness. Mel feels that many of the patients he sees have shown tremendous courage in their lives in trying to cope, and his capacity to perceive that likely contributes to his ability to establish a therapeutic bond with them. At the same time, he is not naïve to the fact that drugs and alcohol do represent a temporary solution for patients, and make them feel transiently better and able to get through the day. He knows this makes them reluctant to relinquish the very things that are both helping and hurting. And that's why, as he points out, the average number of visits by a patient to an addiction program is just one.

RAAM is designed to be a low-barrier program for access: no appointment or referral letter is needed. There is no battery of assessment tools but rather an emphasis on the primary problem identified by the patient. RAAM addresses a range of substance use disorders as well as other physical and mental factors that may be fueling these disorders. It operates through a team approach, and in its current incarnation at Women's College Hospital, where Mel has worked since 2012, it includes a nurse, a physician, and two experienced outreach workers—with the emphasis on establishing therapeutic relationships and being pragmatic and action oriented.

About 60 percent of people booked to attend a RAAM clinic show up for their first visit. While that may seem low, it's actually pretty good for help-seeking. People are often ambivalent about giving up drugs or alcohol, sometimes even when a serious crisis has precipitated their ER visit. But after that initial RAAM encounter, the subsequent visit rate is about 75–80 percent, which really emphasizes how powerful that first visit can be.

For RAAM clinics to work there are two challenges. First, the inflow: they must have a strong initial engagement, with people showing up for their first visit and returning for another. Second is managing the outflow: patients must be accepted into family medicine for follow-up. Otherwise the program becomes clogged with existing patients, impairing its capacity to take on new ones, which is how they work, endure, and grow.

Given that RAAM has been around for two decades, the model and its replication have evolved. In Toronto, there are now seven RAAM clinics, six in general hospitals and one in an indigenous health centre. Around Ontario, there are about seventy clinics currently running, with physicians funded by the Ontario Health Insurance Plan (OHIP) and other staff commonly seconded (voluntarily reassigned) part-time from hospitals and community health programs. They also mostly run in borrowed space from institutions and from the community; these are not clinics that generate the kind of revenue that supports expensive rent. There are similar RAAM clinics in British Columbia, Manitoba, Alberta, and Nova Scotia. And yet for many of my colleagues whom I have informally surveyed, their existence is a surprise.

But the unmet need for RAAM clinics persists, and too often people in crisis are offered nothing. Mel sees a need for even earlier initiation of treatment, when people are seen in the ER. That is essential because of the effectiveness and ease of use of newer anti-craving medications, such as buprenorphine; he feels it should be available as the standard of care in all ERs and family medicine offices in Canada, regardless of lingering negative attitudes toward people who present with opioid use disorders. Mel sees people with addictions as the last accepted repository for stigmatizing and discriminating attitudes and behaviours in health care. He notes that in France, family doctors are very comfortable prescribing such medications and have been doing so for a long time.

However, even among the best intentioned in health care, there are different views. Unlike Benedikt, Mel is not enthusiastic about the option of providing opioid users with medically dispensed opioids as a harm-reduction approach to avoid the risks of buying opioids on the street that may be laced with fentanyl or have other impurities. That strategy, he argues, is intended for a hard-core group of opioid users not reached by other approaches. Instead, he advocates for more dissemination of

RAAM clinics, including one that is being set up within a supervised injection site. He notes that programs to distribute opioids to chronic opioid users are very expensive and cumbersome to set up and will serve only a very small number of people. Further, they are distracting from the real issue that the treatment options offered to these individuals are poor, as is the access to rapid engagement and drugs like buprenorphine. This disparity of views between two experts reflects a challenge in finding the right path forward, but these debates are found throughout health care, from screening to treatment. No one has a lock on the truth, and the generation of evidence (and the willingness to challenge assumptions and dogma) is how we inch forward.

But one thing is certain: We must continue to counter the stigma attached to opioid use. Mel worries about a "moral panic" created by the opioid crisis that leads physicians to abandon or refuse the care of people with existing opioid use disorders. It results in significant opioid withdrawal, sending some to the streets to access more—"we're taking a prescription drug problem and making it worse"—which is exactly what happened to Kirk. A tide rushed in with aggressive opioid prescribing, and receded rapidly, leaving patients beached, stranded, and in withdrawal. For Mel, what is needed is not simply a public health response or an addiction medicine response; this problem was generated by the entire health care system, from dentists to orthopedic surgeons, and the whole system needs to respond.

We both recalled the SARS outbreak in 2003, when the entire health care system responded very quickly to a crisis, much as it has done in a more accelerated and comprehensive way in the 2020 pandemic. No one blamed people for contracting SARS, and no one viewed a SARS death as an acceptable statistic, whereas it is all too easy for clinicians to say to patients, "nobody forced you to use opiates." And as Mel looked back on thirty-five years in addiction medicine, he rued the fact that, unlike other areas in health care, the problems faced now are worse than when he started. Back then, there was a small group of heroin users, generally confined to a marginalized and often criminalized subculture, whom he treated with methadone. Now the group of opioid users and victims is large, diverse, and at risk.

If some members of the current generation of physicians have been unwittingly complicit in the evolution of the opioid crisis, there are younger physicians committed to helping patients out of it. But—as is evident from other chapters—limited traditional resources and long waiting lists act as barriers rather than bridges (or, as are sometimes needed, life jackets).

Aislynn Torfason is a senior resident in psychiatry at the University of Toronto who graduated in medicine from the Northern Ontario School of Medicine, a relatively new school with a focus on recruiting from and serving rural communities. The biggest population of expatriate Icelanders (like Aislynn's family) in the world is in Gimli, Manitoba, but Aislynn was born in the town of Churchill, far to the north in the province, with a population of 899 people and an unspecified number of polar bears. She trained originally in nursing and then in medicine, making her multidisciplinary within herself. She is of the new generation of psychiatrists who feel that the ability to understand and treat people with addictions is a core skill rather than an optional subspecialty. As she spoke with me about this, I recalled how for decades the Clarke Institute of Psychiatry in Toronto stood immediately adjacent to the equally renowned Addiction Research Foundation, but neither patient care nor research nor education was shared across these two institutions. All they shared was the world's worst underground parking lot. Care was completely siloed by professional interests rather than by the needs of patients—one of the critical success factors leading to their integration in the creation of the Centre for Addiction and Mental Health in 1998.

Aislynn is also one of those future psychiatrists who love emergency room work, and in her shifts there she had many encounters with people like Kirk in the midst of an opioid use problem—either suffering from intoxication or withdrawal. So when she learned of an initiative to start treatment in the emergency room, rather than telling someone to go to detox or get on a wait list for residential treatment, she was all in. (It's exactly the kind of program that Mel supports.) What has struck her is the broad range of people under the umbrella of opioid use disorders, from eighteen-year-olds to seventy-year-olds, from chaotic to orderly backgrounds, from lawyers to homeless people and everyone in between. What has also made an impression on her is that she sees no "pure" cases of opioid use disorder; there is always an associated psychiatric or medical disorder to be teased apart and addressed if there is to be any hope of help.

While previously there were treatments that could be initiated in the emergency room, such as using a drug for high blood pressure to suppress acute symptoms of opioid withdrawal, this was more about masking than treating the problem. A team of clinicians working in the CAMH emergency room recognized that the needs of these patients were not being met when they showed up in crisis, and the Suboxone treatment project was born. Aislynn joined the team.

Early in the twenty-first century, Suboxone became available in North America. Its principal ingredient is buprenorphine, a drug that partially activates some opioid receptors in the brain and blocks others. It doesn't cause the high that drugs like Percocet and OxyContin can create but rather reduces withdrawal effects from such opioids. Suboxone's other important ingredient is naloxone, the drug that blocks opioid receptors. Naloxone is present to prevent Suboxone from being abused as another street drug, since naloxone reverses the effects of opioids. Naloxone on its own is found in street overdose rescue kits that many first responders now carry and administer.

The use of Suboxone could be a significant step forward in grappling with a national opioid crisis. But we are more likely as Canadians to hear about naloxone on its own as first responders try to rescue someone from an overdose, as opposed to an ongoing treatment for an addiction. Here is how it would work for Kirk if he came to the CAMH emergency room: First, he would have a careful psychiatric and medical evaluation. Then, importantly, it would need to be determined where he is in his substance use journey and whether he has arrived at the point of wanting help; this treatment is not forced upon people. But that is exactly the desperation that has brought Kirk in.

Kirk is offered treatment at a time when his intensity of need and willingness to get help may be at their most pronounced—when he decides to come to the ER. The moment is ripe for intervention but may not last. If he doesn't get help right away, the cravings may lead to his next dose of opioids on the streets and the closed loop of behaviour is perpetuated. The first dose of Suboxone is given when the patient is in opioid withdrawal. If the patient is still intoxicated on opioids, however, he will be kept in the ER until the first signs of withdrawal start to emerge and treatment can start.

What does withdrawal look like? It could be the emergence of a runny nose, goose bumps on the skin, diarrhea, irritability, and cravings—all in all, an uncomfortable, unpleasant state that can drive people to want to use opioids again, even if they originally came in seeking relief from a vicious cycle.

There is a general assumption that people with substance abuse disorders will reject help. In Aislynn's experience, the majority of people offered help accept it. That should be no surprise. These people had lives prior to their opioid dependence. Coming into the ER, those lives are now obscured to those meeting them for the first time—they may be defined and labeled by their problem. "Coming to the ER in the middle of the night is nobody's idea of a fun time," Aislynn noted, "so if they do show up for help, they are usually open to ideas and suggestions for treatment."

After the first dose of Suboxone in the ER, the patient is monitored for any ongoing signs of opioid withdrawal and possibly a second dose is administered. It may mean that Kirk is in the ER for one to two days—not simply for observation of withdrawal and dosing with Suboxone but also for ER staff to begin establishing a therapeutic relationship and demonstrate a willingness to help someone who might otherwise feel written off.

After twenty-four hours in the ER, Kirk is referred to a RAAM clinic that can see people within a couple of days. At this multidisciplinary clinic, the Suboxone prescribing can be continued while Kirk engages in group psychotherapy treatment and even considers the option of residential treatment. Most people need more than Suboxone alone; they need the psychosocial supports and treatments to help them rebuild and resume some control over their lives—whether it is help with housing, employment, relationship issues, or dealing with past traumas. And where disorders like depression or schizophrenia are present, those also require active treatment.

For people like Kirk, engagement in ongoing treatment varies. And relapses do occur, just as they do with many chronic diseases, from heart disease to bowel problems to cancers. This is taken into account.

Thus there are three elements to this approach that are striking: the use of Suboxone as an emergency and ongoing treatment, the rapid engagement of someone into treatment, and a meaningful multidisciplinary approach to help.

This approach is not simply an ethos; it is a standardized protocol. That means that there is consistency and evaluation built in as a defined "care pathway," while still allowing for flexibility and personalizing the treatment to the needs of the patient. But it also means that it can be exported and scaled up. This is increasingly the approach taken in health care to ensure that people get the same quality of evidence-based treatments regardless of where they are or other barriers. (We have the same protocols for treating the same cancer in different jurisdictions.) Standardized rating scales are used to gauge severity of opioid withdrawal rather than clinical hunches, another example of measurement-based care to guide treatment; dosing of Suboxone is determined by an order set where ratings drive the timing and size of doses. This is very much in the spirit of how the former Addiction Research Foundation set world standards decades ago for measuring and treating people in alcohol withdrawal.

Further, the culture in the ER has changed as a result of this standardized protocol. Clinicians can easily feel helpless in the face of a patient struggling with an addiction; they are unsure of what to do and they bemoan the lack of adequate community resources. Having the evidence-based Suboxone protocol and the RAAM clinic in place allows patients to get help and gives the clinicians confidence and comfort that they can indeed "do something."

The reality is that clinicians can feel frustrated by, and even angry at, people like Kirk. It can be hard to accept that people choose to take an illicit drug, and the fact of it can trigger a negative reaction among health care providers. No one feels that someone "chooses" to have schizophrenia. Aislynn believes a sense of helplessness is at the root of the anger. People go into health care professions driven by a wish to help people. When they feel powerless and inadequate in that regard, anger can emerge as a way of protecting themselves from the reality that they don't have all the answers.

For Aislynn, the biggest surprise of being involved in the Suboxone protocol was how many people were willing and open to being enrolled in it. It challenged her own assumptions—which likely means it also challenged those of people like Kirk.

The CAMH ER is unique in Canada by virtue of its dedication exclusively to people with mental health and substance use disorders 24/7, as opposed to general hospital ERs where people go with problems ranging from dizziness to motor vehicle accident trauma to everything in between (including mental illness and addictions). Indeed, this Suboxone protocol was initiated by physicians at Women's College Hospital in Toronto and run through the ER at several general hospitals. This already speaks to the potential for scaling up. Most people with opioid use disorders who need emergency services will go to a general hospital, so it is essential that the Suboxone protocol be available to them there.

Indeed, Aislynn could imagine this protocol being city-wide, province-wide, and even nationwide. Even at this early stage in her career, she can think of various ERs she's worked in, and the people with opioid use disorders she saw, and wonder, what if the Suboxone protocol had been in place to offer them immediate help? It has impressed upon her that the ER does not need to be simply a waiting room for the queue to get help but rather a place where help is actually initiated. And that's what patients are looking for. Some hospitals have started patients on Suboxone in the ER, but not necessarily in a standardized way.

Despite her enthusiasm, Aislynn doesn't see the opioid crisis ending anytime soon. But she also feels that mental illness and addiction often come as a parcel, and that psychiatry needs to step up and contribute more. She emphasizes that the centrality of building rapport with patients as an essential skill in her training is hugely important in dealing with people with addictions, especially when they are ambivalent about help.

Change needs to happen at multiple levels—how doctors are trained to treat pain, how pain medications are advertised and monitored, and how people who have become addicted to pain medications are helped. While injecting naloxone can acutely bring someone who has overdosed back from the brink of death, and while rapid access to addictions treatments can be a powerful turning point in someone's life, there remain a number of people who are addicted beyond their control or desire to change who face daily risk of death. For them, help may ultimately come from changes in policy and public health. What will it take to end stigma for people like Kirk and to deliver effective and timely treatment? Everyone has a role to play.

8

◇◇◇◇◇

LUKAS AND HOMELESSNESS

IMMEDIATE HOUSING

◇◇◇◇

First Things First

This wasn't supposed to happen. Lukas is more familiar with the shelters of downtown Toronto than he wants to be, as well as the Out of the Cold programs, run by a network of churches and synagogues. He knows where the grates are next to office buildings and over subway lines in the downtown core, where heat wafts up to warm his sleeping bag in winter. Street patrols and police officers know Lukas, bringing him fresh socks or soup, trying to cajole him to consider alternatives to the street, or simply making sure he is alive. An empty paper coffee cup sits near his huddled form, beside a cardboard sign asking for help. Most people walk past Lukas purposefully, not making eye contact and sometimes even accelerating to avoid him. An occasional pedestrian stops, drops some change in his cup, and exchanges a few words. Lukas always responds appreciatively.

At age twenty-seven, Lukas has been on the streets for almost five years. Like every homeless person, there is a backstory as to how he got there.

He grew up in a family with six siblings in northern Ontario, where his father worked as an underground miner and his mother as a grocery store clerk. Mine closures meant unsteady income. Lukas's father's alcohol abuse didn't help matters. He was not a quiet drunk; when intoxicated, he yelled and hit his wife, his children, and unwitting strangers, too. The Children's Aid Society was a frequent visitor to their home, and by the time Lukas was twelve, he had been placed in foster care twice.

Lukas's own alcohol use began at age fourteen and soon evolved to using cannabis, ecstasy, crystal meth, and cocaine. Whether it was the drugs and alcohol or simply bad luck, Lukas gradually developed delusions and hallucinations and in the midst of psychotic fury, he caused a ruckus in a donut shop. He was arrested and charged, his first in a series of encounters with the law that further reduced the chances of him finding work. Failing to appear in court on previous charges compounded his list of legal problems.

He came to Toronto for a fresh start, only to find himself unable to navigate the maze of help resources—social assistance, emotional support, housing, and employment. He found the shelters scarier than the street and discovered the hidden network of other homeless people, as well as those support workers dedicated to trying to help them. But he never felt completely safe or secure, and drugs and alcohol numbed for a moment the fear, as well as the pain that would hit him with every vivid recollection of a childhood filled with physical abuse and threats.

His paranoia led him to trust no one, and to view benign events through a malignant lens. He saw doctors and nurses as part of a conspiracy linked to the government and the Royal Canadian Mounted Police, and he regularly destroyed his documentation to protect himself from their reaches. When a well-meaning street volunteer asked him how he saw his future, he gazed around at the small grocery cart next to his sleeping bag, filled with his belongings, and said plainly, "This."

◇◇◇◇

Every major urban centre in Canada—as well as an increasing number of smaller communities—knows a story like Lukas's; every one of us has walked past a homeless person. And even if you don't see them, it does not mean there is no homelessness problem. All too often, the homeless are tucked away out of everyday sight, temporarily in a shelter, a hospital emergency room, or a jail—all places no one would choose when imagining a place for one's own. Across Canada, it is estimated up to 200,000 people are homeless—more people than the entire population of St. John's, Newfoundland.

For the majority of people who are homeless, mental illness and/or substance abuse have coloured their lives at some point, usually without effective treatment. Homelessness is an expensive problem for Canada, even though the costs are not immediately visible. A sophisticated economic analysis in 2017 of almost 1,000 homeless Canadians with mental illnesses demonstrated that the annual comprehensive costs, excluding any medications, were on average $56,000 per year in Canada's three largest cities based on health, social, and justice services. And that spending does not lead necessarily to improved health and quality of life. Many of them remain homeless.

The immediate solutions seem obvious: feed a person who is hungry, provide a roof and warmth for someone who is sleeping outdoors. Thus the food bank efforts grow and the calls for more shelter beds are ceaseless. But these are finger-in-the-dyke solutions that buy another day, another night, another meal. They do not address either the upstream causes or the downstream consequences of being on the streets in a wealthy nation that prides itself on supposedly universal access to health care and a social safety net. And when homelessness is compounded by mental illness, the traditional approaches to the latter—a scheduled appointment, a prescription, and a treatment program—are usually beyond the reach of someone whose geography for the next twenty-four hours may be completely uncharted.

The pathways to homelessness reflect numerous social, economic, psychological, and physical adversities and misfortunes. These factors are complex, and preventing them from sentencing a person to a life on the streets is a long-term struggle. Meanwhile, we have people freezing, suffering, and dying, right now. No one is actually in favour of homelessness as a social policy or personal outcome. So what can be done?

Part of the answer, at least, can be found in the world's single largest action research on homelessness and mental illness ever conducted. And it was done in Canada. At the same time, very few Canadians seem to know about it. A famous statistician and engineer, W. Edwards Deming, once stated that "in God we trust; all others must bring data." That's what Canada did.

In 2007, the federal government established the Mental Health Commission of Canada (MHCC), thus enacting one of the principal recommendations from a comprehensive Senate report on the current state of mental illness in Canada. That report, titled "Out of the Shadows at Last," was the most extensive examination of the current state of mental illness in Canada in more than half a century. I served as an advisor to the Senate committee, co-chaired by Senators Michael Kirby and Wilbert Keon (a celebrated cardiac surgeon), both during its years of researching and preparing the report, and when the MHCC was enacted, with Kirby as its chair. I became one of its vice chairs, along with Madeleine Dion-Stout, a highly regarded nurse, educator, administrator, speaker, and indigenous advocate.

Within six months of the creation of the MHCC, fortune smiled on the program. Just prior to the global financial crisis of 2008, Canada was fiscally flush. The minister of finance, the late Jim Flaherty, offered a substantial grant to the MHCC in order to conduct a groundbreaking, transformative study. The funding came from government coffers; the big idea on how to use it to advance knowledge came from the MHCC.

A small group of people, led by the late Paula Goering, a PhD nurse (and colleague in my hospital) with expertise in health systems, designed a study to evaluate a solution for homelessness beyond shelters,

ERs, and jails. And thus the study, called "At Home/Chez Soi," was born, with a budget of $110 million—an unprecedented amount in mental health research and in health research in general. It was to be the crowning and final achievement of Paula's distinguished career.

The big question this study asked is, would providing homeless people who have mental illnesses with furnished housing, with rent support and regular visits from a research team member, be better than the existing and sincere efforts to help people with no fixed address and significant mental health needs? The housing would be provided immediately, and given before providing anything else, such as enrollment in formal mental health, substance use, or employment programs. The immediate housing was the experimental arm of the study. To compare it to what would usually be done to help such individuals (the "care as usual" arm), people who participated were randomly assigned to one group or the other. No one could choose which arm to enter, because that's how science uses random assignment to figure out what works better. It may sound like a callous roll of the dice to decide who gets what, but everybody who took part got something and knowledge was advanced.

For Lukas, receiving these new supports would have been a chance to get something more enduring than a hot coffee, a new sleeping bag, and encouragement to come inside during a February cold blast—although in the moment those latter options gave more immediate, if transient, relief. Living at an actual address rather than on the curb of an intersection could potentially provide a more reliable place for Lukas to begin the journey of reintegrating into care for his illness and into a social network. Ultimately it could lead him to a measure of dignity and a more hopeful future.

The experimental arm was an approach known as "Housing First." Importantly, it gave people a choice of housing options and locations almost immediately. The apartments offered were largely private-market units scattered across the five cities—Vancouver, Winnipeg, Toronto, Montreal, and Moncton—where the study was run. Participants on social assistance had to give 30 percent of their monthly income to rent, with subsidies from the study covering the rest of the cost. They had to agree to weekly visits for two years, but not necessarily to treatment or sobriety. After all, how are you supposed to get better—including getting clean and sober—without a roof over your head? Nevertheless, treatments from a team of mental health professionals were available in varying levels of intensity based on clinical need.

More than two thousand people who were homeless and dealing with mental illness were recruited, largely from the streets and from shelters, to take part in the study. That alone was an extraordinary achievement and a tribute to both the participants and the frontline staff of the study who worked to build trust with people who had many reasons to be suspicious. And these were not people who had just recently fallen on hard times. Participants had, on average, been homeless for just under five years. Convincing someone who is living under a bridge, surrounded by plastic bags of their worldly possessions, to trust a stranger who offers them participation in a scientific experiment to end homelessness is no easy feat.

While the average person taking part in the study was a male in his forties, one-third of participants were women, one-fifth were indigenous, and one-quarter were from non-Caucasian ethnoracial groups. More than half of them had not completed high school. All of them had severe mental illnesses, were living in extreme poverty, and more than 90 percent also had a chronic physical health problem.

Toward the beginning of the study, I visited a warehouse in Winnipeg stocked with fresh bedding, sheets, towels, microwaves, utensils, and other necessities—an apartment in a box—that could be loaded into a truck quickly and delivered to an apartment where one of the Housing First participants had chosen to move in. It was a promising sight.

But more inspiring and moving than trips to the warehouses were the visits that I made to participants' new homes, where they proudly agreed to welcome me into their spaces—simple, modest, and clean—and tell me about the profound impact that housing had on their lives. It was a watershed moment that inspired many of the study participants to engage in treatment for the first time, to tackle their substance use, and in some cases to reconnect with family and seek meaningful employment.

Running a complex study like this, working with unique and vulnerable people across five Canadian cities, simultaneously required a large and coordinated local and national effort, led by the MHCC. Each city had unique characteristics: Vancouver's Downtown East Side with its substance use problems; Winnipeg's significant indigenous community, who are overrepresented among the homeless; Toronto's large population and prominent ethnoracial mix; Montreal's long-standing approach to health and social housing for its diverse population; and Moncton's dilemma as a smaller city with a rapidly growing homeless population that includes a rural influx. This allowed for a finer-grain look at how the same approach worked for different jurisdictions and populations, while also generating national data to see how this solution worked for Canada as a whole.

Within each city, coalitions were formed that included clinicians, social service agencies, academics, indigenous and ethnoracial community organizations, and landlords. Many of them were working together for the first time, all around a common goal. Each group and city had its own unique research questions and clinical concerns about local priorities and approaches, but the broader mission was to help solve homelessness at a national level. It was a good blend of one-size-fits-all and what-matters-here.

Dr. Vicky Stergiopoulos, a psychiatrist and researcher, was one of the principal investigators for the Toronto site of At Home/Chez Soi. At the time, she was working at St. Michael's Hospital, an institution dedicated to addressing the needs of inner-city residents, many of whom are precariously housed or homeless. Vicky had first come to Canada at age eighteen from Greece, completing her university and postgraduate education here before returning to Greece. She came back to Canada a second time and enrolled in medical school at Dalhousie University in Halifax, where my father, Richard Goldbloom, taught her in pediatrics. She applied for residency in psychiatry in Toronto and recalls that I interviewed her for acceptance into the program, an encounter I don't remember. She served as psychiatrist-in-chief at St. Michael's Hospital from 2011 to 2016 and then became psychiatrist-in-chief at CAMH—in other words, my boss and the third successor to the job I held fifteen years earlier.

She encountered in her training a population she had not worked with previously: people who were homeless, marginalized in multiple ways, and stigmatized. "I fell in love with the work and the opportunity to make a change," she told me. She began doing community psychiatry that involved working in the shelter system and was mentored by Paula Goering, who engaged her in At Home/Chez Soi. Vicky does not reflect a popular cultural caricature of what it is to be a psychiatrist. She is deeply committed to a disadvantaged and marginalized population— and equally dedicated to marshalling scientific evidence to reinforce advocacy for social justice. She has coauthored many papers about the findings of this major study; her participation in it was a transformative experience for her, a once-in-a-lifetime opportunity to be part of a study that remains globally the leading study in solutions to homelessness.

It still comes as news to many Canadians that we have conducted the world's largest action research study on homelessness, even though it has been celebrated and copied internationally. But while size matters, results matter more. There have been many dozens of scientific papers published based on the program's data, but the big messages for the citizens of Canada (who funded the study) are simple: it can rapidly end homelessness for a significant number of people, and it works in cities that differ in size and composition. That's a big win.

A substantial majority of people in Housing First, many of whom had spent the previous five years in homelessness, remained stably housed after two years. That's a huge change in anyone's life. It significantly outperforms treatment as usual, which for many homeless people still means no help at all. Housing First showed that giving the most vulnerable people in our cities a place to live is not only the right thing to do, but the smart thing, too. At the end of two years, every $10 invested in Housing First resulted in an average savings of $21.72. More fine-grain recent economic analyses continue to mine this unprecedented set of data to understand what works best and for whom. You might have to invest up front in the housing subsidies and treatment services, but there is a financial payoff over time in doing so—not to mention the priceless element of promoting human dignity.

And it's not just about providing housing; most people who were housed were also engaged in treatment and support services. Their quality of life and functioning in the community measurably improved. And the closer that programs adhered to the blueprint of Housing First, the better the outcomes.

The late Jim Flaherty not only oversaw the infusion of money from the government to the MHCC that made At Home/Chez Soi possible; he also tracked its initial findings and chose to translate it into further funding to tackle homelessness outside the study. As minister of finance, he was preparing his 2013 spring federal budget when I met with him in my role as chair of the MHCC. My goal was to share with him the outcomes from the study, and as someone with a keen personal and political commitment to the lives of people with disabilities, he listened intently. It was clear that he saw the return on investment. In his budget, he announced a renewed financial commitment of $600 million over five years to the Homelessness Partnering Strategy, based on the Housing First model. It must be a Canadian record for the journey from idea to research to funding, policy, and action (at least in the era prior to the pandemic).

But it still is not happening fast enough for Lukas and others for whom the streets are home. For far too many of them, the standard of care is simply no care at all. For others, it may be police intervention, incarceration, involuntary hospitalization, or a shelter stay. While these can make a difference, they can often be more expensive and less enduring than going the route of providing housing as a very first step. And the evidence shows that housing-first policy can be a pathway into getting help for a mental illness and getting a better life.

In 2020, new clinical guidelines appeared in the *Canadian Medical Association Journal* for the care of homeless and vulnerably housed people and people with lived homelessness experience—because not everyone is on the streets forever. It is an acknowledgment by the medical profession that this is an underserved, at-risk population whose physical and mental health is broadly determined by social, financial, and physical factors. It identified as priority-need interventions the provision of permanent supportive housing, income assistance, case management, drug treatments for opioid use disorder, and harm reduction efforts for supervised consumption of drugs and management of alcohol problems.

Beyond the long-standing problem of homelessness, the arrival of the pandemic in 2020 brought new challenges to people with severe mental illnesses living in shelters and on the streets. My colleagues at CAMH summarized the implications of COVID-19 for people with schizophrenia and related illnesses. Physical distancing is all but impossible in crowded living arrangements (shelters, jails) and alleyways. People who are psychotic may have more trouble adhering to guidelines around personal hygiene or isolation if needed. They are also more likely to have coexisting physical illnesses that increase their risk to complications of the virus as well as being far more likely to smoke cigarettes than the general population. Finally, they are less likely to seek and to receive medical care for physical conditions. Even before COVID, multiple studies confirmed that people with psychotic disorders die on average twenty years earlier of medical illnesses than the general population. When psychotic disorders coexist with substance use disorders, which is not uncommon, lack of access to care for either set of problems can exacerbate the other. The pandemic only heightens the urgency of the need for solutions to homelessness, and At Home/Chez Soi demonstrates one way this can be achieved.

But there are barriers with an innovation like the Housing First initiative at the core of At Home/Chez Soi, and Vicky Stergiopoulos readily acknowledged this. It is a potential threat to a well-intentioned and hardworking status quo with regard to existing housing initiatives and shelters. And of course when acute crises emerge in relation to homelessness, there is often an immediate need to create new shelter spaces. But, as we have seen in other chapters, more of the same is not always the optimal solution and we need to make more substantive evidence-based changes. And things are never easy. It is important that as a good innovation is scaled up there is fidelity to the model, so that we avoid any dilution of the innovation into something that bears only a passing resemblance to what was proven to work. "Housing First" could become a buzzword as much as "mindfulness" and used for marketing as much as for substance. Finally, when the At Home/Chez Soi study was running, it featured central control to ensure sites were adhering to the protocols, and local variation to reflect unique features or needs of the region. In the wake of the study, there is no single "czar" of homelessness policy and initiatives for Canada, despite it being a national problem. But we do have the Canadian Alliance to End Homelessness, a national coalition of individuals, organizations, and communities with a plainly stated mission: to prevent and end homelessness in Canada. In 2020, this alliance launched its blueprint for a plan intended to end homelessness in Canada by 2030—an ambitious goal, and a worthy one.

This approach, like so many of the innovations described in this book, provides made-in-Canada evidence of what is possible. And like other innovations, it shows the value of something that is not yet accessible to everyone who needs it. We know that it works. We know that it is worth the investment. So, what will it take?

◇◇◇◇◇

CONCLUSION

WE CAN DO BETTER

◇◇◇◇

Canada is far from standing still on mental health. In contrast to two decades ago, the subject is on the platform of every political party, on the agenda of schools and workplaces, and increasingly part of the conversation among all Canadians. We are moving forward, but we are not sprinting, and the finish line is not yet visible beyond the bend in the road. The reality is that this is a relay race over a great distance and the teams involve many people—policy makers, funders, clinicians, researchers, teachers, advocates, patients, families, and friends.

A core aspect of clinical mental health care is, and always will be, talking with and listening to people with the goal of understanding and helping them. The COVID-19 pandemic has forced change upon all aspects of society, and while there remains uncertainty about "the new normal," there is growing consensus it will look different than the old one. The physical distancing and working-from-home guidelines have already transformed what seems normal. At my hospital, televideo assessment and treatment before the pandemic already allowed us to connect with 3,000 patients per year from more than 550 communities across Ontario where access to psychiatry is otherwise poor; I have been part of this initiative for many years and have found it a very gratifying experience. However, a survey of Ontario psychiatrists in 2017 showed that only 7 percent of them participated in this form of care delivery. In February 2020, just before the pandemic restrictions were in place, 327 televideo patient appointments occurred at CAMH. Two months later, there were 3,000 such appointments *per month*—not simply to northern communities but also to downtown Toronto. We are all televideo psychiatrists now.

This is an example not of innovation as much as scaling up an existing and validated but underused approach. The reality is that the first published use of televideo psychiatry to overcome barriers like geography and lack of resources appeared in the scientific literature in 1957. It took a pandemic to force this practice into wider use. Is *that* what it takes?

Of course, mental health needs more money. It's hard to think of a health cause that is overfunded, but Canada beats other countries, such as Australia and the United Kingdom, in a dubious way: it spends a lower percentage of its health dollars on mental health than those (and other) jurisdictions. In 2012, the Mental Health Commission of Canada, in its national mental health strategy, called for the country to increase its mental health spending from 7 percent to 9 percent of all health dollars by 2022; that date is quickly approaching but the increase in spending is not.

At the same time, more money to do more of the same will not be enough. It will not get Shobha or Kirk the help they need, because there are barriers beyond money and limits to the effectiveness of existing services and treatments, even when they are available.

This tour through innovation in mental health, both within Canada and abroad, is not exhaustive. It is also by design not a rigorously comprehensive overview or even a random sample of everything innovative that is currently happening in Canadian mental health. It is a personal journey through things that have caught my attention, aroused my curiosity, and given me hope. One of the advantages of working in a major academic health sciences centre such as CAMH is the opportunity to interact with highly committed clinicians and researchers who are trying to make things better. And if it seems like I have a suspiciously high frequency of personal relationships with them, it reflects my interest in what excites them professionally and my inherent drive for social connection.

Some readers may quibble with the effectiveness of new approaches (nothing in health care works for everyone) and others may balk at which innovations were not included. The longer arc of innovation includes the reality that some shiny new things lose their lustre with time and further evaluation. As my pediatrician father has always said of standards of care, "Today's dogma is tomorrow's malpractice." A more decidedly Canadian approach would have been to consult nationally on what should be included and to ensure that every region and perspective was reflected. From my vantage points as a psychiatrist at the Centre for Addiction and Mental Health, as former chair of the Mental Health Commission of Canada, and as a student of the evolving literature of what works and what's new, I have selected examples driven by the pressing clinical cases I described.

The goal of this book wasn't to be encyclopedic but rather encouraging: there is ample reason that we do not have to settle for the status quo. As things are, too many people in need and their families receive less help than they deserve and less than the evidence suggests could make a difference. And as we've seen, sometimes the status quo means people receive no help at all.

The innovations extend from better use of our genetic makeup to reorganization of how we conceptualize and deliver services—and everything in between. It is not that all we are doing now is wrong—far from it. But it is not enough to meet the need and it is not leveraging enough new knowledge, values, evidence, and technology to achieve real transformation. The good news is that some of this innovation is happening in Canada, even if it has not yet been scaled up to be available to help all Canadians. And Canada has a history of innovation, from Pablum to peanut butter, alkaline batteries to pagers, insulin to pacemakers, Robertson screwdrivers to snow blowers.

If we look at health causes like breast cancer and HIV, public demand for better and newer approaches has made a difference. And Canada has innovated in health care before, from biological advances to health service delivery reform, to stigma busting and peer support promotion. And now the pandemic has made a difference, too—not only in compounding human suffering but also in raising expectations for speed and investment in innovation. In mental health, simply waiting for governments to act will be like *Waiting for Godot*. Innovation needs to be supported, championed, communicated, and scaled up. We can do this.

Notes

◇◇◇◇

INTRODUCTION

9   *It has been argued*: H. C. Wijeysundera et al., "Achieving quality indicator benchmarks and potential impact on coronary heart disease mortality," *Canadian Journal of Cardiology* 27, no. 6 (2011): 756–62.

10 *Another important element has been measuring change*: C. C. Lewis et al., "Implementing measurement-based care in behavioral health: A review," *JAMA Psychiatry* 76, no. 3 (2019): 324–35.

11 *It has been estimated*: Z. S. Morris et al., "The answer is 17 years, what is the question: Understanding time lags in translational research," *Journal of the Royal Society of Medicine* 104 (2011): 510–20.

13 *The first hints*: L. Kang et al., "The mental health of medical workers in Wuhan, China dealing with the 2019 novel coronavirus," *Lancet Psychiatry* 7 (2020): e14.

13 *By March, a review of the evidence*: S. K. Brooks et al., "The psychological impact of quarantine and how to reduce it: Rapid review of the evidence," *The Lancet* 395 (2020): 1–9.

14 *at least one group has identified the risk*: M. A. Reger et al., "Suicide mortality and coronavirus disease 2019—a perfect storm?" *JAMA Psychiatry*, published online April 20, 2020.

14 *In July 2020*: Morneau Shepell, "The Mental Health Index Report Canada July 2020," https://www.morneaushepell.com/sites/default/files/assetspara graphs/resource-list/canadaenglishjuly2020final.pdf.

14 *In August 2020*: Deloitte, "Uncovering the hidden iceberg: Why the human impact of COVID-19 could be a third crisis," https://www2.deloitte.com/ca/en/pages/about-deloitte/articles/crisis-covid-19-human-impacts.html.

14 *Finally, a survey*: R. D. Williams et al., "Do Americans face greater mental health and economic consequences from COVID-19? Comparing the US with other high-income countries," Commonwealth Fund, August 2020, https://doi.org/10.26099/w81v-7659.

CHAPTER 1:
PIERRE AND ATTENTION DEFICIT HYPERACTIVITY DISORDER
(Remote Coaching)

21 *"According to the . . . CADDRA guidelines"*: Canadian ADHD Resource Alliance (CADDRA): Canadian ADHD Practice Guidelines, Fourth Edition, Toronto; CADDRA, 2018, https://www.caddra.ca/wp-content/uploads/CADDRA-Guidelines-4th-Edition_-Feb2018.pdf.

21 *In 2014, a careful review*: G. V. Polanczyk et al., "ADHD prevalence estimates across three decades: An updated systematic review and meta-regression analysis," *International Journal of Epidemiology* 43 (2014): 434–42.

23 *We know from studies of psychiatrist supply*: P. Kurdyak et al., "Universal coverage without universal access: A study of psychiatrist supply and practice patterns in Ontario," *Open Medicine* 8 (2014): e81–e93.

24 *One such program*: Strongest Families Institute website, https://strongestfamilies.com/. P. Lingley-Pottie and P. McGrath, "Imagine a mental health service that delivers stronger families," *Paediatrics and Child Health* 21 (2016): 247–48; J. V. Olthuis et al., "Distance-delivered parent training for childhood disruptive behavior disorder (Strongest Families): A randomized controlled trial and economic analysis," *Journal of Abnormal Child Psychology* 46 (2018): 1613–29; A. Sourander et al., "Two-year follow-up of internet and telephone assisted parent training for disruptive behavior at age 4," *Journal of the American Academy of Child and Adolescent Psychiatry* 57 (2018): 658–68.

CHAPTER 2:
SHOBHA AND ANXIETY
(Integrated Youth Services)

46 *And that was the impetus*: ACCESS Open Minds website, accessopen minds.ca.

46 *The AOM project*: D. Goldbloom, "ACCESS Open Minds/Esprits Ouverts: A seismic shift in Canadian mental health care," *Early Intervention in Psychiatry* 13 , no. S1 (2019): 12–13; S. N. Iyer et al., "A minimum evaluation protocol and step-wedged cluster randomized trial of ACCESS Open Minds, a large Canadian youth mental health services transformation project," *BMC Psychiatry* 19 (2019): 273, https://doi.org/10.1186/s12888 -019-2232-2; A. Malla et al., "Canadian response to need for transformation of youth mental health services: ACCESS Open Minds," *Early Intervention in Psychiatry* 13 , no. S1 (2019): 697–706.

50 *In parallel and in the wake of*: T. Halsall et al., "Trends in mental health system transformation: Integrating youth services within the Canadian context," *Healthcare Management Forum* 32 (2019): 51–55.

51 *Headspace*: https://headspace.org.au/.

52 *But there is reason for hope*: D. Hutt-MacLeod et al., "Eskasoni First Nation's transformation of youth mental healthcare," *Early Intervention in Psychiatry* 13 , no. S1 (2019): 42–47.

56 *For AOM across Canada*: Ashok Malla, personal communication, May 6, 2020.

57 *By the fall of 2020*: Ashok Malla and Srividya Iyer, personal communication, September 16, 2020.

58 *Today Eric is the*: www.jack.org.

CHAPTER 3:
ELYSE AND BORDERLINE PERSONALITY DISORDER
(Short-Term Treatment)

68 *This challenges traditional beliefs*: J. Paris, *Overdiagnosis in Psychiatry: How Modern Psychiatry Lost Its Way While Creating a Diagnosis for All of Life's Misfortunes*, 2nd ed. (New York: Oxford University Press, 2020); J. Paris, *Treatment of Borderline Personality Disorder*, 2nd edition (New York: Guilford Press, 2020); J. Paris, *Stepped Care for Borderline Personality Disorder* (New York: Academic Press, 2017).

70 *In the long journey*: L. Laporte et al., "Clinical outcomes of a stepped care program for borderline personality disorder," *Personality and Mental Health* 12 (2018): 252–64.

71 *It was rigorously evaluated*: S. McMain et al., "A randomized trial of dialectical behavior therapy versus general psychiatric management for borderline personality disorder," *American Journal of Psychiatry* 166 (2009): 1365–74.

72 *Throughout his long career*: J. Paris, "Access to psychotherapy for people with personality disorders," *Personality and Mental Health* 14 (2020): 246–53.

73 *There are more than ten thousand*: M. T. Minen et al., "The functionality, evidence and privacy issues around smartphone apps for the top neuropsychiatric conditions," *Journal of Neuropsychiatry and Clinical Neuroscience* (2020), https://doi.org/10.1176/appi.neuropsych.19120353; K. Huckvale et al., "Smartphone apps for the treatment of mental health conditions: Status and considerations," *Current Opinion in Psychology* 26 (2020): 1–6.

74 *Machine learning has a limitless*: D. T. Hogarty et al., "Artificial intelligence in dermatology—where we are and the way to the future: A review," *American Journal of Clinical Dermatology* 21 (2020): 41–47; X. Du-Harper et al., "What is AI? Applications of artificial intelligence to dermatology," *British Journal of Dermatology* (2020), https://doi.org/10.1111/bjd.18880 online ahead of print.

75 *A well-trained*: D. Dobbs, "The Smartphone Psychiatrist," *The Atlantic*, July/August 2017, https://www.theatlantic.com/magazine/archive/2017/07/the-smartphone-psychiatrist/528726/.

75 *He made a further professional pivot*: www.nesthealth.io.

75 *This has been influenced*: Mental Health Commission of Canada, Newfoundland and Labrador Stepped Care 2.0 e-mental health demonstration project, Ottawa, 2019, www.mentalhealthcommission.ca.

76 *That app may*: A. L. Henry et al., "Insomnia as a mediating therapeutic target for depressive symptoms: A sub-analysis of participant data from two large randomized controlled trials of a digital sleep intervention," *Journal of Sleep Research*, 2020, https://onlinelibrary.wiley.com/doi/epdf/10.1111/jsr.13140.

76 *Meanwhile, in 2020*: F. Matcham et al., "Remote assessment of disease and relapse in major depressive disorder (RADAR-MDD): A multi-centre

prospective cohort study protocol," *BMC Psychiatry*, 2019, https://bmc psychiatry.biomedcentral.com/track/pdf/10.1186/s12888-019-2049-z.

78 *It is currently a bit of a Wild West*: U. Ebner-Priemer et al., "Digital phenotyping: Hype or hope?" *Lancet Psychiatry* 7 (2020): 297–99; N. Lau et al., "Android and iPhone Mobile Apps for Psychosocial Wellness and Stress Management: Systematic Search in App Stores and Literature Review," *Journal of Medical Internet Research* 8, no. 5 (May 22, 2020): e17798, https://doi.org/10.2196/17798.

79 *A 2019 study*: K. Huckvale et al., "Assessment of the data sharing and privacy practices of smartphone apps for depression and smoking cessation," *JAMA Network Open* 2, no. 4 (2019): e192542.

80 *Recent careful research*: K. Huckvale et al., "Smartphone apps for the treatment of mental health conditions: Status and considerations," *Current Opinion in Psychology* 36 (2020): 1–6; M. T. Minen, "The functionality, evidence and privacy issues around smartphone apps for the top neuropsychiatric conditions," *Journal of Neuropsychiatry and Clinical Neuroscience* (2020), https://doi.org/10.1176/appi.neuropsych.19120353.

80 *In 2020, a survey*: A. R. Wasil et al., "Examining the reach of smartphone apps for depression and anxiety," *American Journal of Psychiatry* 177 (2020): 464–66.

82 *And in the United Kingdom*: B. Inkster et al., "An Empathy-Driven, Conversational Artificial Intelligence Agent (Wysa) for Digital Mental Well-Being: Real-World Data Evaluation Mixed-Methods Study," *Journal of Medical Internet Research mHealth and uHealth* 6, no. 11 (2018): e12106.

82 *And it is the first in its class*: K. K. Fitzpatrick et al., "Delivering cognitive behavior therapy to young adults with symptoms of depression and anxiety using a fully automated conversational agent (Woebot): A randomized controlled trial," *Journal of Medical Internet Research Mental Health* 4, no. 2 (2017): e19.

83 *Despite the potential*: A. Baumel et al., "Objective user engagement with mental health apps: Systematic search and panel-based usage analysis," *Journal of Medical Internet Research* 21, no. 9 (2019): e14567, https://doi .org/10.2196/14567.

83 *As one of the world experts*: J. Linardon et al., "The efficacy of app-supported smartphone interventions for mental health problems: A meta-analysis of randomized controlled trials," *World Psychiatry* 18 (2019): 325–36.

84 *It is challenging for clinicians*: https://www.psychiatry.org/psychiatrists/practice/mental-health-apps.

84 *And a recent randomized*: A. K. Graham et al., "Coached mobile app platform for the treatment of depression and anxiety among primary care patients: A randomized clinical trial," *JAMA Psychiatry* 77 (2020): 906–14.

85 *Mental Health Commission of Canada*: P. McGrath et al., "Toolkit for e-Mental Health Implementation," Mental Health Commission of Canada, Ottawa, ON, 2018, https://www.mentalhealthcommission.ca/sites/default/files/2018-09/E_Mental_Health_Implementation_Toolkit_2018_eng.pdf.

Chapter 4:
Richard and Panic Disorder
(Self-referral)

92 *A national survey*: Angus Reid Institute, "Worry, gratitude & boredom: As COVID-19 affects mental, financial health, who fares better; who is worse?" http://angusreid.org/covid19-mental-health/.

93 *There, in an office*: https://www.england.nhs.uk/mental-health/adults/iapt/.

93 *IAPT began in England*: R. Layard and D. Clark, *Thrive: The Power of Evidence-Based Psychological Therapy* (London: Penguin, 2015).

94 *Within a year*: D. Clark, "Realizing the mass public benefit of evidence-based psychological therapies: The IAPT program," *Annual Review of Psychology* 14 (2018): 159–83.

94 *The IAPT Manual*: The National Collaborating Centre for Mental Health, "The Improving Access to Psychological Treatments Manual," version 4, 2020, https://www.england.nhs.uk/wp-content/uploads/2020/05/iapt-manual-v4.pdf.

99 *BEACON is a web-delivered*: www.mindbeacon.com.

101 *Of course, those results*: P. Farvolden et al., "Beyond mild-to-moderate symptoms: Therapist-assisted iCBT by BEACON® is effective for more severe symptoms of generalized anxiety," Toronto, MindBeacon Health, 2020 (report available from MindBeacon Health on demand).

101 *But these evolving*: E. P. Stech et al., "Internet-delivered cognitive behavioral therapy for panic disorder with or without agoraphobia: A systematic review and meta-analysis," *Cognitive Behavior Therapy* 49 (2020): 270–93; C. Luo et al., "A comparison of electronically delivered and face to

face cognitive behavioural therapies in depressive disorders: A systematic review and meta-analysis," *EClinical Medicine* 24 (2020): 100442, https://www.thelancet.com/journals/eclinm/article/PIIS2589-5370(20)30186-3/fulltext; E. Axelsson et al., "Effect of internet vs face-to-face cognitive behavior therapy for health anxiety: A randomized noninferiority clinical trial," *JAMA Psychiatry*, May 2020, https://doi.org/10.1001/jamapsychiatry.2020.0940; R. Buscher et al., "Internet-based cognitive behavioral therapy to reduce suicidal ideation: A systematic review and meta-analysis," *JAMA Network Open* 3, no. 4 (2020): e203933, https://doi.org/10.1001/jamanetworkopen.2020.3933; M. Baumann et al., "Cost-utility of internet-based cognitive behavioral therapy in unipolar depression: A Markov model simulation," *Applied Health Economics and Health Policy* 18 (2020): 567–78; M. E. Thase et al., "Improving the efficiency of psychotherapy for depression: Computer-assisted versus standard CBT," *American Journal of Psychiatry* 175 (2018): 242–50.

103 *That was the experience of Bell Canada*: Deloitte Insights, "The ROI in workplace mental health programs: Good for people, good for business," Toronto, 2019, https://www2.deloitte.com/ca/en/pages/about-deloitte/articles/mental-health-roi.html?nc=1.

CHAPTER 5:
MARTHA AND DEPRESSION
(Personalized Care)

112 *When the World Economic Forum*: World Economic Forum Global Agenda Council on Workplace Mental Health 2014–2016, "Seven actions towards a mentally healthy organisation," http://www.joinmq.org/pages/seven-actions-towards-a-mentally-healthy-organisation.

112 *And beyond this particular program*: Resilience@Law Legal Profession Mental Health Toolkit, 2020, http://www.blackdoginstitute.org.au/wp-content/uploads/2020/04/black-dog-institute-mental-health-toolkit-resilience@law.pdf?sfvrsn=2&sfvrsn=2.

113 *Indeed, when in 2013*: Mental Health Commission of Canada, National Standard of Canada for Psychological Health and Safety in the Workplace, 2013, https://www.mentalhealthcommission.ca/English/what-we-do/workplace/national-standard.

115 *But the chances*: B. N. Gaynes et al., "What did STAR*D teach us? Results

from a large-scale, practical, clinical trial for patients with depression," *Psychiatric Services* 60 (2009): 1439–45.

116 *The accounting firm Deloitte*: Deloitte, "The ROI in workplace mental health programs: Good for people, good for business," 2019, https://www2.deloitte.com/ca/en/pages/about-deloitte/articles/mental-health-roi.html?nc=1.

117 *Currently, fewer than 20 percent*: C. C. Lewis et al., "Implementing measurement-based care in behavioral health: A review," *JAMA Psychiatry* 76 (2019): 324–35.

117 *However, researchers have also identified*: E. H. Connors et al., "What gets measured gets done: How mental health agencies can leverage measurement-based care for better patient care, clinician supports, and administrative goals," *Administration and Policy in Mental Health and Mental Health Services Research* (2020), https://doi.org/10.1007/s10488-020-01063-w.

118 *This is the essence of personalized medicine*: E. B. Quinlan et al., "Identifying biological markers for improved precision medicine in psychiatry," *Molecular Psychiatry* 25 (2020): 243–53.

120 *A 2014 study*: J. Fagerness et al., "Pharmacogenetic-guided psychiatric intervention associated with increased adherence and cost savings," *American Journal of Managed Care* (2014): e146–e156.

120 *A major American randomized*: M. E. Thase et al., "Impact of pharmacogenomics on clinical outcomes for patients taking medications with gene-drug interactions in a randomized controlled trial," *Journal of Clinical Psychiatry* 80, no. 6 (2019): 19m12910.

121 *And a 2019 review*: C. A. Bousman et al., "Pharmacogenetic tests and depressive symptom remission: A meta-analysis of randomized controlled trials," *Pharmacogenomics* 20 (2019): 37–47.

121 *In Canada, a 2020 review*: A. Al Maruf et al., "Pharmacogenetic testing options relevant to psychiatry in Canada," *Canadian Journal of Psychiatry* 65 (2020): 521–30.

121 *At least one modeling study*: J. A. Tanner et al., "Cost-effectiveness of combinatorial pharmacogenomic testing for depression from the Canadian public payer perspective," *Pharmacogenomics* (2020), https://doi.org/10.2217/pgs-2020-0012.

122 *The costs for each test*: C. Lunenburg et al., "Pharmacogenetics in psychiatric care, a call for uptake of available applications," *Psychiatry Research* 292 (2020), https://doi.org/10.1016/j.psychres.2020.113336.

123 *Lucky for us*: S. Sehatzadeh et al., "Unilateral and bilateral repetitive transcranial magnetic stimulation for treatment-resistant depression: A meta-analysis of randomized controlled trials over 2 decades," *Journal of Psychiatry and Neuroscience* 44 (2019): 151–63; D. M. Blumberger et al., "Effectiveness of theta burst versus high-frequency repetitive transcranial magnetic stimulation in patients with depression (THREE-D): A randomised non-inferiority trial," *The Lancet* 391 (2018): 1683–92; E. J. Cole et al., "Stanford accelerated intelligent neuromodulation therapy for treatment-resistant depression," *American Journal of Psychiatry* (2020), https://doi.org/10.1176/appi.ajp.2019.19070720.

124 *That's a failure of advocacy*: K. P. Fitzgibbon et al., "Cost-utility analysis of electroconvulsive therapy and repetitive transcranial magnetic stimulation for treatment-resistant depression in Ontario," *Canadian Journal of Psychiatry* 65 (2020): 164–73.

124 *As Cassius says to Brutus*: D. S. Goldbloom and D. Gratzer, "Barriers to brain stimulation therapies for treatment-resistant depression: Beyond cost-effectiveness," *Canadian Journal of Psychiatry* 65 (2020): 193–95.

125 *In 2018, a major Canadian study*: Blumberger et al., "Effectiveness of theta burst."

125 *The next year*: A. B. Mendlowitz et al., "Implementation of intermittent theta burst stimulation compared to conventional repetitive transcranial magnetic stimulation in patients with treatment resistant depression: A cost analysis," *PLoS ONE* 14, no. 9 (2019): e0222546, https://doi.org/10.1371/journal.pone.0222546.

125 *More Canadian evidence in 2020*: Fitzgibbon et al., "Cost-utility analysis of electroconvulsive therapy."

CHAPTER 6:

MANUEL AND SCHIZOPHRENIA

(Training as Treatment)

132 *Recent Canadian data*: P. J. Gill et al., "Emergency department as a first contact for mental health problems in children and youth," *Journal of the American Academy of Child and Adolescent Psychiatry* 56 (2017): 475–82.

132 *There are some national*: https://epicanada.org/.

135 *Sean has a particular interest*: S. R. McGurk et al., "A meta-analysis of cognitive remediation in schizophrenia," *American Journal of Psychiatry*

164 (2007): 1791–1802; E. R. Revell et al., "A systematic review and meta-analysis of cognitive remediation in early schizophrenia," *Schizophrenia Research* 168 (2015): 213–22; L. Morin et al., "Rehabilitation interventions to promote recovery from schizophrenia: A systematic review," *Frontiers in Psychiatry* 8 (2017), https://doi.org/10.3389/fpsyt.2017.00100.

136 *No, which is a shame*: S. A. Kidd et al., "Cognitive remediation for individuals with psychosis in a supported education setting: A randomized controlled trial," *Schizophrenia Research* 157 (2014): 90–98.

136 *Sean, like most experts*: "Schizophrenia in Canada: The social and economic case for a collaborative model of care,": Public Policy Forum, Ottawa, ON, 2013, https://ppforum.ca/wp-content/uploads/2018/03/Schizophrenia-in-Canada-Final-report.pdf.

136 *If CR is designed*: S. A. Kidd et al., "Testing a modification of cognitive adaptation training: Streamlining the model for broader implementation," *Schizophrenia Research* 156 (2014): 46–50; S. A. Kidd et al., "A pilot study of a family cognitive adaptation training guide for individuals with schizophrenia," *Psychiatric Rehabilitation Journal* 41 (2018): 109–17.

138 *This technology, called*: S. A. Kidd et al., "Feasibility and outcomes of a multi-function mobile health approach for the schizophrenia spectrum: App4Independence (A4i)," *PLoS One* (2019), https://doi.org/10.1371/journal.pone.0219491.

140 *It is easy to imagine*: M. Knapp et al., "Associations between negative symptoms, service use patterns, and costs in patients with schizophrenia in five European countries," *Clinical Neuropsychiatry* 5 (2008): 195–2005.

142 *Using a VR task*: J. A. Zawadski et al., "Simulating real world functioning in schizophrenia using a naturalistic city environment and single-trial, goal-directed navigation," *Frontiers in Behavioral Neuroscience* 7 (2013): 1–10.

143 *The potential benefits*: M. Rus-Kalafell et al., "Virtual reality in the assessment and treatment of psychosis: A systematic review of its utility, acceptability and effectiveness," *Psychological Medicine* 48 (2018): 362–91; K. Gainsford et al., "Transforming treatments for schizophrenia: Virtual reality, brain stimulation and social cognition," *Psychiatry Research* 288 (2020), https://doi.org/10.1016/j.psychres.2020.112974.

CHAPTER 7
KIRK AND OPIOID USE DISORDER
(Multidisciplinary Approach)

150 *The term "deaths of despair"*: A. Case and A. Deaton, *Deaths of Despair and the Future of Capitalism* (Princeton, NJ: Princeton University Press, 2020).

151 *Based on three different rates*: S. Petterson et al., "Projected deaths of despair during the coronavirus recession," Well Being Trust, May 8, 2020, https://wellbeingtrust.org/wp-content/uploads/2020/05/WBT_Deaths-of-Despair_COVID-19-FINAL-FINAL.pdf.

151 *At the same time, there is*: Y. Bao et al., "COVID-19 could change the way we respond to the opioid crisis—for the better," *Psychiatric Services* (2020), https://doi.org/10.1176/appi.ps.202000226.

151 *In Ontario*: T. Gomes et al., "Measuring the burden of opioid-related mortality in Ontario, Canada," *Journal of Addiction Medicine* 12 (2018): 418–19.

152 *In Canada, between*: B. Fischer et al., "Crude estimates of prescription opioid-related misuse and use disorder populations towards informing intervention system need in Canada," *Drug and Alcohol Dependence* 189 (2018): 76–79; B. Fischer et al., "The opioid death crisis in Canada: Crucial lessons for public health," *Lancet Public Health* 4 (2019): e81–e82.

153 *The missing piece*: M. Tyndall, "A safer drug supply: A pragmatic and ethical response to the overdose crisis," *Canadian Medical Association Journal* 192 (2020): e986–987, https://doi.org/10.1503/cmaj.201618.

154 *At the same time*: "Prosecution of Possession of Controlled Substances Contrary to s. 4(1) of the *Controlled Drugs and Substances Act*," Public Prosecution Service of Canada, https://www.ppsc-sppc.gc.ca/eng/pub/fpsd-sfpg/fps-sfp/tpd/p5/ch13.html.

155 *the limits to existing*: M. R. Krauz et al., "Been there, done that: Lessons from Vancouver's efforts to stem the tide of overdose deaths," *Canadian Journal of Psychiatry* 65 (2020): 377–80.

158 *But the unmet need*: A. Srivastava et al., "Buprenorphine in the emergency department: Randomized clinical controlled trial of clonidine versus buprenorphine for the treatment of opioid withdrawal," *Canadian Family Physician* 65 (2019): e214–e220.

168 *It has impressed upon her:* K. F. Hawk et al., "Barriers and facilitators to clinician readiness to provide emergency department–initiated buprenorphine," *JAMA Network Open* 3, no. 5 (2020): e204561, https://doi.org/10.1001/jamanetworkopen.2020.4561.

CHAPTER 8
LUKAS AND HOMELESSNESS
(Immediate Housing)

171 *A sophisticated economic analysis:* E. A. Latimer et al., "Costs of services for homeless people with mental illness in 5 Canadian cities: A large prospective follow-up study," *CMAJ Open* 5 (2017): e576–e585.

172 *That report, titled:* Standing Senate Committee on Social Affairs, Science and Technology, "Out of the Shadows at Last: Transforming Mental Health, Mental Illness and Addiction Services in Canada, Ottawa, 2006."

173 *It was to be the crowning:* P. Goering et al., *National At Home/Chez Soi Final Report* (Calgary, AB): Mental Health Commission of Canada, 2014, https://www.mentalhealthcommission.ca/sites/default/files/mhcc_at_home_report_national_cross-site_eng_2_0.pdf.

176 *That's a big win:* V. Stergiopoulos et al., "Effect of scattered-site housing using rent supplements and intensive case management on housing stability among homeless adults with mental illness: A randomized trial," *JAMA* 313 (2015): 905–15; T. Aubrey et al., "A multiple-city RCT of Housing First with assertive community treatment for homeless Canadians with serious mental illness," *Psychiatric Services* 67 (2016): 275–81

177 *More fine-grain recent economic analyses:* E. A. Latimer et al., "Cost-effectiveness of Housing First with assertive community treatment: Results from the Canadian At Home/Chez Soi trial," *Psychiatric Services* (2020), https://doi.org/10.1176/appi.ps.202000029.

178 *In 2020, new clinical guidelines:* K. Pottie et al., "Clinical guideline for homeless and vulnerably housed people, and people with lived homelessness experience," *Canadian Medical Association Journal* 192 (2020): e240–254, https://doi.org/10.1503/cmaj.190777.

178 *My colleagues at CAMH:* N. Kozloff et al., "The COVID-19 global pandemic: Implications for people with schizophrenia and related disorders," *Schizophrenia Bulletin* 46 (2020): 752–57.

179 *But we do have:* www.caeh.ca.

179 *In 2020, this alliance*: S. Pomeroy, "Recovery for All: Strategies to Strengthen the National Housing Policy and End Homelessness," Canadian Alliance to End Homelessness, 2020, https://www.recoveryforall.ca/report.

CONCLUSION:
WE CAN DO BETTER

184 *However, a survey*: E. Serhal et al., "Implementation and utilisation of tele-psychiatry in Ontario: A population-based study," *Canadian Journal of Psychiatry* 62 (2017): 716–25.

184 *The reality is that*: H. Tucker et al., "Television therapy: Effectiveness of closed-circuit television as a medium for therapy in treatment of the mentally ill," *AMA Archives of Neurology and Psychiatry* 77 (1957): 57–69.

Acknowledgments

◇◇◇◇

In 2016, Simon & Schuster Canada took a chance on two rookie authors—academic psychiatrists by day and aspiring writers by night—in publishing *How Can I Help?: A Week in My Life as a Psychiatrist*, co-written with my colleague Pier Bryden. The response from readers, both the general public and health professionals, was heartwarming and encouraging. In the wake of that experience, Kevin Hanson, the president and publisher of Simon & Schuster, asked me what I would like to write about next. He emphasized his commitment to the subject of mental health. For that encouragement and leadership, I am forever grateful.

However, I assumed Kevin did not want me to write about a second week in my professional life. That book had reflected both current clinical practice and its historical roots. This time I wanted to focus on the future, with the goal of providing hope as well as information about innovation. But I also wanted to keep it anchored to the reality of the challenges people face today and to ask how things could be better, not a generation from now, but a couple of years from now.

The answers were not immediately in my head but rather in the heads and actions of others. Every one of the innovators I interviewed for this book gave generously of his or her time, including responding to my endless "me again" emails and phone calls to clarify and update their contributions. My profound thanks goes to them not only for sharing their work and enthusiasm but also for doing their work in the first place. They have enriched the mental health landscape. And my good fortune in working at the Centre for Addiction and Mental Health and the University of Toronto means that I count some of these innovators as my longtime colleagues and friends.

It is an unfortunate reality that a book about innovation becomes dated by the time of publication. It is not an impulsive tweet but a considered and refined reflection. However, given the lag time between discovery and implementation, I hope that the innovations described remain both surprising and encouraging to readers.

The other reality is that books like this are selective rather than encyclopedic. I know many colleagues in Canada and elsewhere who are doing innovative things not described in this book. To those not included in this "tasting menu," I apologize and thank you for the important work you do.

With our previous book, the experience of working with a literary editor proved to be an epiphany and a humbling graduate seminar in how to write. As much as I gleaned from that experience, writing this book took me further down that learning path, ably guided initially by Brendan May and subsequently at greater length by Justin Stoller. Their suggestions, questions, and edits both illuminated concealed points and deflated bloated prose. Our margin comments exchanges would make a hilarious separate—and at times tasteless—book. But in the end I remain in awe of their talents and their preferential empathy for readers over authors!

My literary agent, Michael Levine, has been a relentless cheerleader and advocate in this journey, fusing his deep knowledge with a genuine passion for mental health. His guidance and support have been invaluable to me.

For writers with a day job doing something else, stolen moments are needed after-hours to create a book. Many evenings following dinner with Nancy, my wife of forty-five years, I have gone to my study to "do my homework"—reading about innovations, writing about them, and responding to the high tides of red ink from Justin's computer on what I had assumed was a polished masterpiece. While those hours of solitude were necessary, the reward has always been rejoining her afterward, the person for whom I am most grateful in life.

Acknowledgments usually include the statement that while multiple people made the book possible, any errors, inaccuracies, or omissions are the sole responsibility of the author. It is with great reluctance that I accept that accountability.

Index